Advice
and
Info
to Get
Teens
in the
Know

Am I Weird or Is This Normal?

Marlin S. Potash, Ed.D., and Laura Potash Fruitman
with Lisa Sussman

A Fireside Book
Published by Simon & Schuster
New York London Toronto Sydney Singapore

FIRESIDE
Rockefeller Center
1230 Avenue of the Americas
New York, NY 10020

FIRESIDE and colophon are registered trademarks
of Simon & Schuster Inc.

Designed by Joy O'Meara
Illustrations by Susanne Saenger

Manufactured in the United States of America

1   3   5   7   9   10   8   6   4   2

Library of Congress Cataloging-in-Publication Data

Potash, Marlin S.
Am I weird or is this normal? : advice and info to get teens in the
know / Marlin Potash and Laura Potash Fruitman with Lisa Sussman.
p. cm.
Includes index.
1. Adolescence.   2. Teenagers—Life skills guides.   3. Interpersonal relations
in adolescence.   4. Puberty.   5. Sex instruction for teenagers.
I. Fruitman, Laura Potash, 1984–   II. Sussman, Lisa, 1961–   III. Title.
HQ798 .P67 2001
305.235—dc21   2001033219

ISBN 0-7432-1087-5

MEDICAL DISCLAIMER

This publication contains the opinions and ideas of its author. It is intended to provide helpful and informative material on the subjects addressed in the publication.
It is sold with the understanding that the author and publisher are not engaged in
rendering medical, health, psychological, or any other kind of personal professional
services in the book. If the reader requires personal medical, health, or other assistance or advice, a competent professional should be consulted.

The author and publisher specifically disclaim all responsibility for any liability,
loss, or risk, personal or otherwise, which is incurred as a consequence, directly or
indirectly, of the use and application of any of the contents of this book.

We dedicate this book to Perle and Monroe Potash—
may we always make you proud

Acknowledgments

This book could not have been written without the help of our wonderful editor, Doris Cooper, who shepherded it with good humor all the way; invaluable input from Hilary Potash Fruitman, our unofficial third author (we thought you were too young to be our co-author when we started writing and you proved us wrong!); the patience of Steven, Jazz, and Tasha; and the insight of our agent, Todd Shuster.

Various professionals and organizations ensured that our information was accurate and up-to-date. We gratefully thank William Pollack, Ph.D., for his *Real Boys* and belief in our vision to help real girls; and Kathleen Cowan, who earned our admiration for reading the whole shebang in its rawest stage and giving us helpful notes. Also, eternal gratitude to Frank Petito, M.D., the professional colleague everyone should be so lucky to have in their corner. A special thanks to Amy Beecher for her terrific illustrations in Chapter 3, and to Bob Stein, who helped us edit the "must-keep" from the "gotta-go."

Thanks to David Burgreen, Ben Diskant, Chris Fisher-Lochhead, Hannah Frank, Colleen Hall, Rachel Heyman, Dan Manso, Ben Preston-Fridman, Rachel Rosenberg, Matt Schneier, Nic van der Meer, and to the entire class of 2002 at Friends Seminary in Manhattan: You've all been a great help with everything! Particular thanks go to David Arnold, former head of Upper School at Friends Seminary, and all the Upper Schoolers there, who were so generous with their time, energy, and ideas about adolescence.

Appreciation to Fiamma Arditi, Mary Pipher, Norine Johnson, Ph.D., Ronald Levant, Ed.D., The Hon. Sheila E. McGovern, Alfred Mendelsohn, Wendy Oppenheim, Kary Presten, Burt Rosenberg, John Sahag, and Sarah Snider for their unique contributions and inspiration along the way.

With gratitude to Planned Parenthood; Youth Crisis Hotline; Step Family Foundation; Women's Sport Foundation; Girls Incorporated; Students Against Destructive Decisions (SADD); Anxiety Disorders Association of America; Parents, Families and Friends of Lesbians and Gays (PFLAG); National STD Hotline; National Clearinghouse for Alcohol and Drug Information; National Domestic Violence Hotline; Rape, Abuse & Incest National Network (RAINN); National Eating Disorders Organization.

And to all the patients and friends who shared their stories about adolescence so that our readers could benefit. We hope they, too, have benefited by the reliving and rethinking. We know our readers will be as enriched by their generous sharing as we have been.

Acknowledgments

Contents

The Life List

You're smart.
You're funny.
You're beautiful.
You're strong.
You're a nice person.
You're interesting.

So why do you feel so nervous, scared, dorky—so *weird* compared to everyone else?

We want you to know that *everyone* thinks: "I'm a freak. I'm different. I'm weird!" Even the most popular girl, the most self-assured girl. First, there's the weirdness that happens when you feel out of it because you've grown breasts and no one else has, or you're the only one wearing a skirt to a party where everyone else has the new in-jeans. Then there are the times when you desperately want to fit in and worry that every word out of your mouth sounds weird.

Sometimes you're weird because of circumstances beyond your control—like the color of your skin or the size of your nose or your sexuality. Doesn't matter.

One of the reasons we wrote this book? We think weird is normal. Everyone feels that they are different. In our house, calling someone "weird" means acknowledging someone who is her own person, who

11

believes what she wants, and who has the courage to express herself in that special way that no one else can copy.

We wrote this book to help you deal with your own particular brand of weirdness. So that after reading it, you'll be able to say, "Okay, yeah, I'm weird—and that's totally normal."

Your parents' rules make you feel like a 10-year-old.

You argue with your friends about new and intense issues like who is popular, who stuffs, who has a boyfriend, who is having sex, who uses drugs, where to hang out.

You feel pressure at school where, if you flub one math test, you worry about not getting into a good college.

And you feel the world at large bombarding you with wild ideas and images of the "typical teen," as if there were such a thing.

To top it off, the pressures that probably hit hardest are those you put on yourself.

To help you get on solid ground and zap away that nagging, insecure feeling, consider what we call the *Life List,* a map for dealing.

The rest of this book is packed with facts, explanations, ideas, and stuff to help you make your own decisions, but the Life List has 16 guidelines to carry with you, like your house keys and lip stuff. Don't memorize them—this is no algebra exam. Just keep them handy.

1. Believe It

If you act like you think you're okay, everyone else will believe it, too. No one is born with confidence, but everyone can develop it.

It may sometimes seem there are voices inside you or around you trying to wear you down. Answer those voices when they call you lame. Take away their power by reminding yourself of your talents: You are someone who can tell a joke, run fast, play the guitar, decorate your room—whatever it is that you have confidence in. Borrow it from yourself.

Now put your new (even if it feels fake) "believe it" image out into the world. Just like an actor, play a part and make your voice strong, express your opinions with gusto, and walk tall with your shoulders back.

If you project the strength you wish for, you will absorb it, like osmosis.

If you think it's okay to sit at the lunch table alone, then it is. If you want to wear baggy clothes and be hip-hop, go ahead. If you'd rather stay home Saturday night and write poems, do it. If you decide it's okay, then it is. That's the point.

2. Shout It Out

You hear a lot about expressing yourself but not much about how to do it. Shouting it out can make you feel like a player in your own life. Keeping quiet makes you feel smaller and weaker, less entitled and more depressed, as if your thoughts and words were less deserving than everyone else's.

Girls are often more quiet than boys because they lose self-confidence when they become self-conscious about their bodies changing. Girls deal with growing breasts, which are obvious, but boys don't have to deal in a public way with the size of their penises (although they do worry).

Also, society sends a "shush" message. TV shows, song lyrics, movie plots, magazine articles, even teachers and family often suggest that girls should just be seen, not heard. As a result, you may worry about making waves, looking silly, or being embarrassed about how you might sound, all of which makes it easier to keep your mouth shut. But feeling and acting as if you have a right to say what you think changes how other people look at you.

Here are some ways to shout it out:

- Chime in when friends are deciding where to go out. Chances are they will welcome the suggestion.
- Say something when your date is always late. Show him you deserve respect.

13

- Raise your hand in class when you know the answer. Why not let the teacher know how on top of it you are?
- Talk to your parents about their rules. You'll have an opportunity to convince them that you are responsible. You might not get everything you want, but you won't get anything without asking.

3. Stand Out and Be Someone

Don't be afraid to be yourself. It's tempting to look for refuge in cliques, gangs, and groups. But acting a certain way just to impress people always does anything but. And when you act in a way that's comfortable, people look up to you.

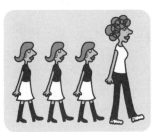

When you set your own trends, the rest of the world may eventually catch up. Think Rosie O'Donnell, Shannon "Mac" MacMillan, Lisa Loeb. An overweight talk-show hostess sensation, a soccer player with big thighs, a dorky-looking singer. These women are all different and they flaunt their personal signatures and strengths. They have come out on top by *not* compromising who they are.

Here are some big and small ways to stand out and be someone.

- Wear your hair in braids.
- Start a club at school.
- Begin a conversation with someone in your school who you've never talked to before.
- Be the first girl on the all-male wrestling team.

4. Reach Out and Make Friends

Friends can help you deal with anything: shaving, crushes, loneliness, and every emotion ever invented. True friends will grow with you.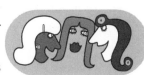

If you choose well, here are some things reaching out and making new friends can do for you:

- Keep you company
- Show you new things you might not find on your own
- Encourage you
- Clarify decisions by taking the pro when you take the con, and vice versa

Keep an open mind about who could be a friend. Choose people who make you feel good about yourself. Their social status shouldn't be part of the equation.

5. Rule It

Try to stay cool and in control.

There will always be situations that get you fired up. And times when you are going to feel angry or just plain bitchy. But you can control the invasion of feelings so that they don't run your life.

Here's how to rule it:

Think of situations that have made you lose it (your parents wouldn't let you go to a party, your friends pushed you to smoke a joint, a teacher picked on you). Now think: What did those moments have in common? Did you feel you couldn't have what you wanted?

Once you do this, you will know what gets to you, and you can be on the lookout for that one thing that gets you going. You don't want the same old responses to keep happening to you—you want *you* to control your feelings.

6. Know Your Strengths

Like everybody else, you've got pluses and minuses. Figuring out what they are can make you feel good about yourself because then you can focus on the good and deal with the bad. Don't get so absorbed by the stuff you're not so hot at that you lose the joy you could get from things in which you excel.

To know your strengths, take time to think through what you're good at:

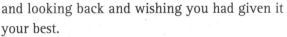

* You write like Maya Angelou.
* You can sink three-point baskets.
* You're a good cook.
* You always do your work on time.

Now think about what you're not so hot at:

* You can't tell an octagon from a hexagon.
* You run slower than a tortoise.
* You have a terrible singing voice.
* You can never remember names.

Update this mental list every month or so. There may be things you used to feel were weaknesses—like being too nice—that you now see as pluses.

7. Take a Risk

Real courage comes from acting even when you are afraid. Regrets and anger with yourself come from not having the courage to try, and looking back and wishing you had given it your best.

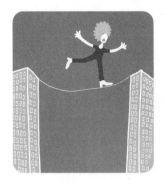

So go ahead and try out for the squad or a part in the play, or ask your crush out on a date, even though you think you're more likely to fail than win. Even if you do fail, at least you didn't pass up the chance and then have to wonder if you could have made it happen. When you succeed, which you will, you'll feel even more powerful and ready to take a risk.

Here are some healthy ways you can take a risk:

* Make a new friend.
* Take a tough class.

🌀 Say no to something you don't believe in even when everyone else is saying yes.

🌀 Join a club where you don't know anyone.

8. Make Anger Work for You!

You can recycle anger. You can take some of the crap in your life and turn it into fertilizer to grow flowers.

In some cases, the energy of being furious may change a situation, but generally there is much that teens and adults alike are powerless to do anything about. So the thing to do is express anger in a positive way.

Your anger can define you positively or negatively. It's up to you to choose: (A) You can act out your rage by the drugs–alcohol–shoplifting–meaningless sex route. You'll get immediate payback that can feel good—at the time. But it doesn't last. *Or* (B) You can say to yourself, "I'm furious, this pisses me off," then move beyond your anger by tackling the reason for it head-on. For instance, a student at McAteer High School in San Francisco, angry about the generally lame energy there, decided she could change her environment. She and a few others formed SPAM (Students for Positive Action). They planted a Peace Garden in an outdoor walkway, lent portable gardens in buckets to a teacher or student having a hard day, collected clothing and food for the homeless, and posted signs asking, "If we don't change the world, who will?"

You can act out your inner wrath and make your anger work for you by:

🌀 Screaming in the shower or turning your music up loud when no one else is home

🌀 Helping others and taking the focus off yourself

🌀 Getting a part-time job to earn your own money so that you feel you have more power in getting some of the things you want

🌀 Talking calmly to whomever you are angry at without making accusations

9. Wear the Other Shoes

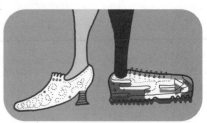

Think how good you feel when someone is sympathetic toward you. Well, sympathy is a get-what-you-give thing. This is especially true when dealing with parents.

Here's how to wear the other shoes:

- ❧ Listen to what the other person is saying rather than acting as if you're listening when you're just waiting long enough to jump in with your side.
- ❧ Remember that someone who doesn't think like you is not necessarily stupid.
- ❧ Keep an open mind—trying on someone else's ideas can put a new slant on your own.

10. Let It Go

Instead of torturing yourself over what's not fair, learn to *accept*. Think of all the time you can waste getting stuck on things you can't change—like your parents' divorce or the fact that you spaced a math test. You probably still won't like the situation, but you won't be wasting energy and beating yourself up.

So, to let it go:

- ❧ Ask yourself if there is anything you can realistically do to change the situation.
- ❧ Listen to yourself and accept the fact if the answer turns out to be no.
- ❧ Remind yourself that what's done is done. You can never go backward in time.

11. Ride It Out

Try to get into the thrill of the whole emotional roller coaster of your life—even the stomach-wrenching turns. Think how you feel about a roller coaster: You wait impatiently in line, excited, eager. Then the ride starts. As the car climbs higher, you have doubts: "Maybe this isn't such a good idea. It's too high, too steep." But you realize you're committed to the experience. There's no backing out now.

Your life may feel like this. One second, you are so excited and so in control that you could conquer the world. The next, you feel totally confused, depressed as hell.

Make your slogan, "What doesn't kill you makes you stronger." This is the only time you'll ever go through all these firsts: first crush, first kiss, first dumped-by-guy-before-you-got-kissed, first boyfriend, first job, first big mistake you'll always regret.

Here's how to enjoy the ride:

- Write down all your roller-coaster experiences in a journal and revisit every few months—you'll see what was once a big deal is now a funny memory or a memorable experience.
- Talk with your friends—the best way to deal with fear is to acknowledge it. Chances are, you'll find out they're going through a lot of the same experiences.

12. Forgive and Forget

Give the world a break. Do your best to get over the ways you've been let down. Your friend is going to blow you off, your parents are going to show how much they don't get you, your boyfriend is going to act dorky, your teacher is not going to give you the grade you deserve, your boss is not going to recognize all your sterling qualities, and the rest of the world is going to ignore you.

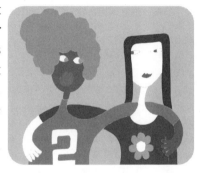

19

So when parents or friends disappoint you, forgive and forget:

🌀 Remind yourself that they love you, they are trying to do their best, and they might still know a thing or two that you don't.
🌀 Tell yourself that imperfect doesn't mean totally wrong.
🌀 Remember, we all blow it a few times along the way (including you). It's the only way to learn to make the right choices next time around.

13. Know Your Limits

When it comes to your life, you really are your own best expert. Plan to be the only one who makes decisions for you.

If you figure out ahead of time what your limits are—what you are and are not prepared to do (as opposed to following what everyone else is doing)—you'll be set to face any high-pressure situation like deciding whether you want to use drugs, get drunk, have sex, ditch a class, or run away from home.

Stop right now and assume that within the next year you're going to be confronted by just about every weird, stressful, uncomfortable scenario on the planet. Now take a piece of paper and answer the following:

🌀 How far do I want this to go? Why?
🌀 How far would I go for a friend? Why?
🌀 How do I feel about doing something my parents have told me not to do? Why?
🌀 How do I feel about breaking the law? Why?
🌀 How do I feel about trying anything once? Why?
🌀 What would I do/say if I didn't want to do everything that everyone else was doing?

Once you know your own answers, you know your limits and you're prepared to deal with anything that comes up.

20

14. Let It Shift

You can always reinvent yourself. Your personality, opinions, goals, even your circle of friends do not have to be set in stone.

Life is constantly changing—doors open, doors close. Just because you did something once doesn't mean you will want to again. Just because you liked something once doesn't mean that you still do (you can outgrow things). Just because you hated something once doesn't mean you won't like it later.

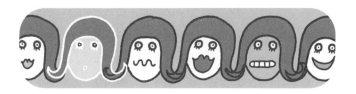

Remember that situations evolve, energy levels vary, and desires change. Here are a few ways to let it shift:

- 🌀 Sign up for a class you never thought you were interested in to learn new things and meet different kinds of people.
- 🌀 Try a food that seems disgusting to you.
- 🌀 Flirt even though you don't think you're good at it.

You will see yourself evolving.

15. Mellow Out

Everything in life has its own potential for stress. You have a boyfriend? You get anxious if he seems distant or starts pressuring you for sex. You have a great group of friends? You think they're not "in" enough (not that you really care, but still . . .).

There are standard stresses: grades, teachers, the future, your parents, acne, your body, just trying to get through the day. This is how you mellow out:

- 🌀 Take a deep breath and push all your tension out with your outer breath. Buddhists call this muting the monkey mind—

21

stifling all the thoughts that clutter your brain so that you can focus on a solution.

- Take a warm bath. A few drops of lavender oil has been shown to help relax the mind.
- Listen to soothing, quiet music.
- Keep a journal. It gives you a chance to vent without blowing up at an unsuspecting friend or family member.
- Read a book or magazine. Reading relaxes the mind and the body.

16. Get Some Perspective

A huge part of being happy comes from gaining perspective. Who you are is so much more than the person who fumbles killer points on the debate team, fails a history test, or can't Rollerblade to save her life.

Take a break from navel-gazing and notice other people's worlds. When you look around, you will realize that others are so preoccupied with their own personal pangs that they aren't even paying attention. If you don't believe that, consider this: How much time do you spend thinking about someone else's bra size? Well, that works both ways.

Take time out to notice what other people are experiencing and do what you can to give them a helping hand. They'll appreciate the effort and you'll also win, because you've stopped directing all your attention and energies toward yourself, if just for one brief moment.

It's easy to see what you *think* you don't have. Get some perspective by realizing what you *do* have:

- Life
- Health
- People who love you
- Talents
- Youth
- Your own personal uniqueness

- A roof over your head
- Enough to eat
- An education
- The freedom to choose (although it may not always feel like it, think about what life would be like if you lived in Bosnia or Iran)
- The opportunity to be whoever and whatever you want

1
Getting It On

How do I meet someone to date?
How do I get someone to go out with me?
What should we do when we're out together?

None of us know intuitively how to tell if someone is interested, or how to deal with the possible rejection, or what to say on a date. These things are learned through trial and error.

Potentially embarrassing? Yes. Because part of the thrill of going out with someone is feeling accepted. It's like winning a People's Choice Award. You feel like jumping up and saying, "He likes me. He really, really likes me!"

But the risks of dating—or trying to get a boyfriend—are much lower if you approach dating not from the attitude of "How can I get someone to go out with me?" but "What do I want from this?"

Never thought of it that way, did you?

This chapter will give you a handle on how to work out the balance between boys and your life without losing your mind.

Crushes

Crushes are bittersweet. They can make your day tolerable.

But one-sided yearning can also be painful. The object of your passion may never give you the time of day. Which is why, ultimately, this state of being is called a crush (as in *demolish),* not a boost.

> I have a crush on this guy at school, and he's all I can think about.

DR. MARLIN: When you have a crush, you think you're in love but you're not. Okay, so you can't stop thinking about the guy and your heart beats a mile a minute when he's near.

But this passion is based on fantasy. After all, what do you really know about this guy other than that he looks good?

Sometimes this sort of fantasy love is much better than the real thing: He's perfect. It's fun to indulge. It's easy to read love signals into his every move. It can even be a confidence booster because you convince yourself he's drooling over you when he really has no interest in you.

Decide if you'd rather stick with the fantasy or if this is something you want to try to make happen. Not all crushes are worth acting on, especially if the person is someone off-limits like your best friend's boyfriend.

Here's how to decide: Do a reality check on your crush, in which you find out at least five true things about him.

Are these qualities you would want in a boyfriend? For instance, if you find out that he dumped his last girlfriend over the phone or that he's always goofing off in class, he may not be right for you.

If it turns out that you are still interested in him, you might want to go for it—gently. If you did your reality-check homework, you have some idea what he's interested in and if it interests you, too. Act on that. Talk to him about whatever you have in common.

LAURA: It's not easy to just approach some guy who you really like, let alone talk to him. You have to connive the situation a little by putting yourself in his path. I really liked this guy who was in another grade, so there was hardly any opportunity for us to connect. Then I found out he was taking an architecture class that I'd been planning to take the following year. So I signed up right away.

Okay, we didn't end up going out. But we did become great friends, which can be another bonus of crushing on a guy.

There are lots of not-so-obvious opportunities to get near him. Hang out at a friend's locker near his, go to the candy store where he goes, or try to get next to him on the lunch line. Eventually make eye contact and say something. If there's the slightest chance he's interested, he'll start talking, even if it's just a grunt. If he's picking up your signals and doesn't send one back, then take the hint and move on.

Getting a Date

In poll after poll, guys say the same thing: They hate fake. In other words, wanting to be in a relationship so desperately that you act in a way that's not you is the number one turnoff. The only thing you can do to make yourself sizzle is to be real. Here's how:

◇ Know you are important with or without a boyfriend. A desperate girl attracts a different kind of attention than a proud one does. Guys, like girls, want to be with winners. A confident girl gives off the aura of worthiness: "I respect myself and expect you will respect me, too."

◇ Don't just agree. And, for God's sake, don't play dumb. When you speak your mind, you stand out as an interesting person. Don't worry if he sees things differently. Guys—well, anyone you'd want, anyway—are attracted to women strong enough to hold to their own opinion.

◇ Stay active. Becoming more involved with things around you—whether sports, mentoring, or art—advertises you as a fun and interesting person. Guys don't want some one-note chick they have to entertain all the time. Hey, would *you*?

◇ Look good. Take a long, honest look at yourself to figure out how to make the best of the features you have—including the physical ones. In other words, don't hide your growing breasts. They're part of what makes you a woman, so stand straight and wear clothes that fit. Instead of hiding behind your hair or trying to disappear behind layers of makeup, get a beauty makeover (free at most department stores) and a haircut that shows off your face. Stop buying into the system by being a fashion victim. Wear shoes and clothes that let you feel comfortable and move like your normal self (see Chapter 4 for instructions on finding your own style).

••

I've never had a date.

••

DR. MARLIN: *Yet.* You've never had a date *yet.* I know. This seems like the same old line and *not yet* usually feels like *never.* However, the main thing isn't to live life looking for a date but to keep on reaching out and making some friends.

The more situations you put yourself in where you are doing things that grab your attention, the more likely you are to connect with people you click with—and that includes the opposite sex.

You don't want to go out with just anyone who asks you. You want someone who is going to be right for you. And the only way to find that person is to do the things you enjoy and stay open to meeting new people.

LAURA: Society still has a way to go to change its expectations of the male making all the date arrangements. But girls aren't hanging around the phone hoping he'll call anymore, either. So instead of holding your breath waiting for some guy to do the asking, why don't you take some risks? Approach someone you're crushing on and pop the question yourself.

I'm not saying it's easy. But lots of guys are shy, too. I know my guy friends hate that they are always expected to make the first move.

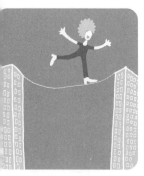

Otherwise, you're saying you'd rather ask yourself "And what if . . ." "If only I had the guts to . . ." So my advice is to just do it and get it over with. Don't make a big deal of it. The best line, according to guys, is, "Wanna do something sometime?" The guy can't panic and blurt out, "Sorry, I'm not free," because you haven't set the time yet. In fact, you haven't even asked him for a date yet! Nothing's official, so if he wants to back out, he can, without leaving either of you feeling too embarrassed.

Check out his reaction, too. If he mutters something about not having any free time for a long time, quit while you're ahead. Simply say something like, "Well, maybe another time," and let it go at that.

Remember, guys get this treatment all the time and bounce back. As one of my guy friends says, "When I get rejected, I can't think it's me, or I'd never ask a girl out again. I just think that it means the girl wasn't right for me and I'm better off without her."

If he doesn't outright reject you, follow up with, "So what do you want to do?"

• •

Boys only see me as a great friend.

• •

DR. MARLIN: This is not necessarily a bad thing. In fact, there's real value in boys seeing you as a friend.

If you're a close friend, you're probably seeing more of your guy friends as their authentic selves than any girlfriend would. It's unlikely that they would be as completely open with her as they are with you because they're trying to impress her (think of how you act around friends versus a guy who *you* like). Also, as their friend, you are developing a strong foundation of trust.

All these things are great precursors to a solid romantic relationship. In fact, many couples in solid relationships say getting to know their partner as a friend before they got romantically involved helped keep them strong as a team because they already had a connection that went beyond sexual attraction.

Flirting Basics

Flirting is good. And it's easy. Effective flirting starts with one simple thing: *Get him talking about himself.* The simple truth is that showing interest by listening is appealing.

Here's how to do it:

⋄ Make eye contact. Not a slow, deliberate gaze from across a crowded room—that's staring, and it's uncomfortable. Hold the other person's gaze and smile. This displays friendliness and self-confidence (even when you don't feel that way yourself), which are the most attractive qualities you can have.

⋄ Start the conversation. Guys rated the following lines as the best icebreakers:

LAURA: Although it may seem like guys only think of you as a friend and can't see you as a potential girlfriend, that might not always be true. If a guy is comfortable around you and likes spending time with you, he may like you and not know it yet (look at Dawson and Joey. It took him a while, but then he fell head over heels). I would also use this time to find out what guys really think about things (like what kind of girl would they like to date vs. hook up with). You can get some great insight that could come in handy with boys that you really like.

Why is it that only the guys I don't like ask me out?

DR. MARLIN: Simple. They're the ones you are able to be most comfortable around because you're not interested in them as potential boyfriends.

Unfortunately, we tend to get more nervous and sweaty when we are

- "Hi."
- "Do you want to dance?"
- "That's a cool shirt."

◇ Expand the conversation by saying a line or two about yourself, such as: "I really love [insert favorite comedian]'s new show." Or " I'm learning to snowboard. It's really different from skiing." This will give the other person a chance to pick up on what you say if he's interested in continuing the conversation.

◇ Check out his look and then use it to get him talking about himself. If he's wearing a football jacket, say, "I heard you had a great game on Saturday." Or if he has some band's stickers all over his book bag, ask him what he thought of their latest single.

near someone we have a crush on because we try so hard. And the guy picks up on that and thinks this is your normal self.

The way around it is to remind yourself that as cute as a boy may be, he is just a boy. Repeat this mantra when you start thinking he's too cool for you: "He's just a guy. Maybe a cute one. Maybe a funny one. Maybe a cool one. But he's just a guy, like I'm just a girl." When you can transform your crush back into human terms, you'll be able to calm down enough to become your regular self.

LAURA'S TIP: One thing that works for me is to remember how I act when I'm with my guy friends just hanging out. Did I tell a joke or story they liked? Then I'll repeat it when I'm with a guy I like.

If you want the guys who you do like to ask you out, try spending time with them as a friend so that you can be really comfortable around them. It may or may not develop into a boyfriend thing. Chances are that the guys who might make better boyfriends are the ones you can talk to naturally rather than always worrying about saying the right thing.

....
I like a boy who isn't cute and I'm afraid my friends will make fun of me if I date him.
....

DR. MARLIN: It's time to take some risks. Never let your desire to fit in stop you from acting on what you want in life (see Chapter 6). After all, real friends want you to be happy.

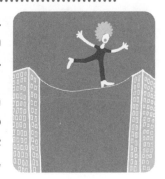

Besides, a boyfriend should never be an accessory—something you wear on your arm to complement the image you want to project. He should be a person you love to spend time with, no matter what other people think.

LAURA: Okay, Mom, but it's still really hard to move outside of your clique. It can make you feel isolated. You don't want to think your friends are talking about you behind your back, and you also want to be able to think that you and your guy and your friends can all hang together without feeling weird.

I'm not saying you shouldn't go for it. But your relationship is going to be under a lot more pressure than most because you will be hyperaware of the criticism.

Sound your friends out on the guy—maybe saying how he seems sort of cute when you look past his height or whatever else they are criticizing. It's easier to change their minds so that they see him in a new light than it is to ignore your own heart.

On a Date

....
I never know what to say on a date.
....

DR. MARLIN: Stand out and be someone. The key is to be yourself. After all, that's who he was attracted to in the first place and that's who he asked out.

Five Dating Don'ts

1. *Don't set unrealistic expectations.* He won't be Brad Pitt or the man of your dreams. He's just a mere mortal—like you. Wish for the best. Expect reality. You won't be disappointed.

2. *Don't be fake.* Don't pretend to like something you don't. It might get him to like you initially, but sooner or later he'll find out and feel betrayed.

3. *Don't deceive him.* If you're not into him, shout it out in a nice but firm way. When you figure out for yourself that it's not going to work, break the news nicely. It'll save loads of heartbreak and wasted time for you both.

4. *Don't ask for too much too soon.* No one wants to feel pressured into love. Let things go at a steady pace.

5. *Don't think chemistry is everything.* It's important, but acting on it too soon will only create discomfort. The best sex requires intimacy, and you can't create intimacy just by having sex.

If you're not sure who that self is, think how you are when you are with your friends or your family. Talk about the same things you would talk about with them.

Say something that will get him talking. Try asking him about himself—his summer plans, how big his family is. This isn't about the male ego dominating the conversation, just getting him to converse so that it's not all on you.

Just don't ask him too many intense questions too soon, tell him your life story in the first 10 minutes, get too heavy about why you're crushing on him, or complain about anything too personal. Guys just aren't comfortable with the same kind of personal conversation that girls usually use as a way of bonding.

LAURA: I always ask questions because that keeps me from talking too much and helps to get him talking. Ask open-ended questions so that he doesn't just grunt a reply. But don't hit him with nonstop questions or you're gonna sound like Ricki Lake.

And if you can't think of any questions to ask him, just pretend that you're talking with your brother or your best guy friend. In other words, act like your normal self.

Getting Serious

....

I like two guys and can't choose.

....

DR. MARLIN: Who says you have to? It's sometimes hard to know whether a guy is for you until you've gone out with him a few times. And even then, you may find there are things you like about one guy and things you like about the other.

I actually think it's a good idea to date more than one guy at a time. Here's why: You refine your taste by getting a sense of what's out there— brains, humor, sensitivity, self-confidence—so you can

Boy Nerves

Boys actually get worse date jitters than girls. A study of 3,800 undergraduates at the University of Arizona found that 37 percent of men compared to 25 percent of women were nervous during a date. That's why so many guys seem to sit there like a mute when you're out with them.

Five All-Purpose Questions to Keep Him Talking

1 Have you ever been here [the setting the two of you are in] before? (Discuss anyone you know who works there.)

2 What's the worst movie you ever saw? Seen any funny movies lately?

3 Are you into [name a sport or activity you like]?

4 What do you think of [name of teacher everyone hates]?

5 If you had to spend a month in the hospital, who would you most like to share the same room with, and why?

decide what qualities are essential to you in a relationship. Think of it as "comparison shopping."

However, it can also be stressful. One or both of the guys may not be so happy with the idea of sharing you and act jealous. This might sound like fun—having a guy get territorial over you—but do you really want to Be asked to account for your every second when you are away from him?

If you think you can handle it, then there are some ground rules: Be straight with yourself and with the guys—they don't have to know about each other, but you do need to inform them that you're not interested in making an exclusive commitment, so that neither thinks he's your only one.

Also, don't: date guys who are friends; overlap them or see them on the same day; gossip about one to the other; go with one where you think the other might be; or date one boy just to make another jealous.

LAURA: I hate the whole you-go-out-with-someone-once-and-now-you-have-a-relationship deal. It's much more fun to hang and see a few guys at once. After all, there's plenty of time in life to get married and settle down.

Don't forget to let it shift. Remember, people change, situations change, attitudes change—sometimes daily. So be open to the possibility that after a few dates you may realize that you prefer one boy to the other or even that you're not crazy about either of them. In which case, do the right thing and let the rejected guy(s) go as gently as you would want to be dropped.

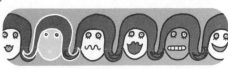

Five Must-Haves for Dating

1 *A good ego.* Have a positive outlook about yourself (and make sure he feels the same).

2 *A level head.* Okay, he's gorgeous. Physical attraction is great, but you have to have things in common and like being with each other.

3 *Patience.* You need to get to know each other before you can call him your boyfriend. A relationship worth having is worth the wait.

4 *Trust.* First, trust yourself. Go for what's best for you and check if he fits those criteria. If so, choose to trust him.

5 *Knowledge.* Know what you want and shout it out. One person shouldn't have to make all the dating decisions.

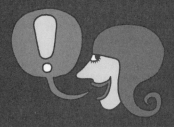

> The guy I like has a girlfriend. He says he loves her, but he keeps flirting with me. Why does he do that?

DR. MARLIN: Because he's confused and doesn't know what he wants, or because he's a two-timing bastard. Either way, let it go. You can talk to him, but I don't think it will do much good. It seems like he will keep on vacillating about what he wants.

I know—if I am such a big fan of going after what you want, why don't I tell you to go for it? Because there are times when you know in your heart of hearts that what you want isn't really good for you in the long run, and it sounds like this is one of them. Let's say he ends up with you. Would you ever really be sure that he wouldn't pull the same stunt with another girl?

LAURA: It sounds to me like he wants you. The guys I know tend to be more up front in what they *do* rather than what they say. So I'd say go for it. But go slowly—just in case he changes his mind again.

> Why would a guy say he's going to call and not?

DR. MARLIN: Guys love saying this. It buys them time to think about their feelings toward you.

It could be that he's afraid to call. He may have forgotten. What you interpreted as a soul connection was a casual flirt for him.

Whatever the reason, just let it go. You can go over it in your head again and again, endlessly discuss it with friends, and still not be able to figure it out.

Bottom line: Any guy who doesn't want to call you is too much work. And dating should be fun, not an exhausting mind game.

LAURA: Not getting a call back sucks. It's happened to me and it used to make me want to wallow in my bed (which would also allow me never to be more than 2 feet from my phone just in case he did call).

If you absolutely must call him for peace of mind, then keep it simple. Call him only once. Just say you're calling to say hi, or to thank him for the excellent time you had with him.

If he acts distant or unenthusiastic, saying something like "I meant to call you" without saying why he hasn't, or, "I can't really talk right now" without mentioning when he can talk, or if you leave a message and he never gets back to you, then at least you know where you stand.

....

A guy who's 8 years older than me asked me out. Is he too old for me?

....

DR. MARLIN: Many girls find older men more attractive and sophisticated than boys their own age. Your body be fully developed by age 12 whereas some boys may not reach full maturity until their early 20s (see Chapter 4).

So you have to ask yourself, "Why is he interested in me?" No matter how talented, interesting, or beautiful you are, his interests and views on life are bound to be different from yours. Chances are he is very immature and/or needs some element of control in the relationship and gets that by going out with someone who is younger and therefore less likely than women his own age to challenge him.

But no matter how mature you are (or how immature he is), the one absolute truth is the bigger the age difference, the bigger the problems. For instance, having sex. He's more likely to be experienced and to expect it as part of the relationship. Fifty percent of girls 15 to 17 who get pregnant are sleeping with a guy who is at least 20.

Also, in some states, where the age of consent is 18, having sex with him could land him in jail for statutory rape—even if you gave your consent.

I'd say give this one a pass.

LAURA: I know all the guys your age seem really stupid. That's because they are. And it can make you feel really cool to go out with a guy who's older.

But a guy who is that much older than you is also probably way ahead of you socially, mentally, sexually, emotionally. He has a whole different life—he can drink legally (if he is 21), get into clubs, get a driving license, and vote. He's not worried about your learner's permit test because he's too busy worrying about college or work.

LAURA'S TIP: *Think*—would you go out with someone 8 years younger than you? Exactly.

One Last Dating Tip from Dr. Marlin

You do not need a guy to feel good about yourself, although it's tempting to go that route. But you do need to feel good about yourself to find a guy who is right for you. So think about the qualities you really care about in a boyfriend. (If you're stuck on what to write, put down qualities that you like in your friends.)

Looks, too, are usually important to us all (let's be honest), but did you ever notice that when you really like someone and you're happy with each other, you look better (and so does he)?

Prioritize your list. All items on your list are not of equal importance. Some are "absolute musts" and others are "would be nice but not a deal breaker." For example, it might be okay if your new boyfriend doesn't care much about mountain biking (even though you're crazy about it), but maybe it's really essential he be a non-smoker.

After you've completed your list, look it over carefully. Is it realistic? (In other words, could any one person possibly have all of those wonderful qualities?)

The point is that the best relationships are based on mutual admiration. If you secretly hope that he will eventually change his style, that's a sign that it might be time to move on to someone you really appreciate for who he is (or vice versa if he pressures you to make all sorts of changes).

If, on the other hand, you feel satisfied and he likes the things about you that you like about yourself, then you're onto something really great.

39

2
Getting Together

You're going to have bad relationships as well as good ones. That's practically a given as you explore the vast variability and potential of love. This doesn't mean you're setting yourself up for a lifetime of love unhappiness. It just means you're learning what you do and don't want from a relationship. Finding perfect love depends not so much on finding the perfect person as on finding someone who is the right kind of imperfect for you. This chapter will help you to start being smart with your heart.

Communication

Does talking with your boyfriend sometimes feel like talking to a brick wall? Figuring out how to talk to each other and even argue with each other can help you achieve a greater sense of well-being and connection with your relationship.

Love Timeline

Real-life relationships breathe—sometimes you feel closer and sometimes you feel more distant. Here's a rough idea of a relationship's average life cycle:

First Week: Pure bliss. You are convinced that you have found the perfect person.

Second Week: Best behavior prevails.

Third Week: Your real life may have fallen by the way-side as you spend all your time together trying to find out everything you can about each other.

Fourth Week: The fog clears. At this point there is a natural drawing back from the intense intimacy of your early days together. Although that time was wonderful, you would smother each other if it went on forever.

First Month: You reconnect with your "before" life (there's nothing worse than a friend who dumps you just because she has a boyfriend).

Second Month: Certain personality "warts" might start to bug you. Remember, people are who they are, and they don't become different unless they want to. So basically what you see is what you get.

Third Month: You're officially a couple. That means you're working out your friends, faults, and interests within your relationship.

Whenever my boyfriend and I fight, he stops speaking to me for days. How can I get him to open up?

DR. MARLIN: So-called grown men do this, too. It's one thing for him to need some breathing time after a fight to clear his head and figure out how to deal. But what he is doing is mean.

First, make sure you're fighting fair: Stick to the issue at hand. Don't lecture, yell, or bring up past hurts. This is hard.

If he still gives you the silent treatment, tell him how it makes you feel (scared it's over, frustrated about what to do). Then ask him what would make it easier for him to talk. He may say he doesn't know. But expressing how you feel means at least he knows it bugs you, and hopefully he will make more of an effort to not shut down in the future.

LAURA: Guys are conditioned from a young age not to reveal their emotions. Sometimes, they don't even know what they're feeling. One study found that both boys and girls smile equally until age 9. Then boys, responding to the tough-guy images they get from TV and movies, begin to shut down because they think it's more masculine.

When I fight with my best guy friend, he always seems to need a "Laura break." Being away from me helps him not to get so mad at me, and when we see each other again after a weekend apart, we're fine. Usually I realize that even though he didn't *say* he was sorry, his actions—calling me after an exam to make sure I feel okay—show how he feels.

So you can talk to him once about how it bothers you, but badgering him and getting him to talk about it is a waste of time and will only make him more mad at you.

DR. MARLIN'S TIP: Screaming matches over small stuff—like what movie to see or forgetting directions—are often actually about big stuff—like the balance of power in your relationship.

What to do? Skip the fight and let it go. How you handle all of these little tussles are what will make or break you as a couple. The thing that makes a solid relationship is realizing you don't always have to be right or even see eye-to-eye.

The next time you're about to blow up over some petty thing—like who should drive—stop and say, "You know, this is a dumb argument. Let's not have it." Then either agree to disagree or compromise—say, "Okay, if this is so important to you, you drive there and I'll drive back."

> My boyfriend is fine when we are alone but acts embarrassed whenever I try to hold his hand in public. Does this mean he doesn't love me?

DR. MARLIN: No, it means he may be shy. Just because guys are the ones who often have to make the first overt move in asking you out or kissing you for the first time doesn't mean that they're never scared or shy. Boys have a macho image that they feel they have to live up to, including never revealing their emotions and acting like they are in control all of the time. Which means if you bring it up, he will probably act defensive and deny that he has a problem.

Instead, show him some consideration and wear the other shoes. The pace of a relationship should always be the pace of the slower person. So try holding his hand at the movies or in the car when you are with friends. If he seems comfortable with that, you can move up to giving him a casual hug or kiss. However, he may never feel comfortable showing affection in public. That may just be his style.

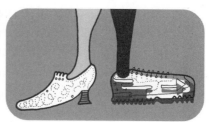

LAURA: I had to call in the guys on this one. A couple of them thought if your boyfriend does it in private but not in public, he may be ashamed of you (and then added that he probably isn't since he's dating you). One—okay, he's a bit of a macho jerk—said he may be afraid of seeming "whipped" or that his friends will think you control him if he acts nice to you. Most said they see PDAs as something private.

And they all said, "Why ask us? Why not ask him? He'll tell her."

Whenever my boyfriend sees a pretty girl, he stares at her—even when he's with me. I've asked him to stop, but he won't. Why does he do this?

DR. MARLIN: The same reason guys like to look at pictures of naked women and movies that have sexual images: Males are hard-wired to respond visually. So they are turned on mostly by things that they see. Women, on the other hand, get aroused by what they hear and feel. Which is why you like to hear him tell you that he loves you and whisper sweet nothings in your ear whereas he would much prefer to just look at you.

So if he is just glancing at other girls, don't take it as a sign of how he feels about you. He is following his instincts. However, if he is actually gawking or looking in such an obvious way that he can't carry on a conversation with you, you have every right to feel insulted.

He needs some behavior modification. Tell him that the next time he starts staring, you are going to leave. Then do it.

You'll need to think ahead on this, as it will mean finding your own way home if he doesn't behave appropriately. But I don't think you will need to do it more than once or twice for him to get the message that his staring is insulting to you and you won't put up with it.

LAURA'S TIP: Excuse me, but he's a boy. Boys are attracted to girls. Just because he's with you doesn't mean he's suddenly supposed to become blind to the existence of other girls. I mean, if you saw Freddie Prinze Jr.'s twin walking down the street, wouldn't you turn your head? I don't think he's going to stop.

Try staring at cute guys in front of him. Let him know how it feels.

> It sometimes seems that if I didn't call my boyfriend to make plans, we'd never see each other.

DR. MARLIN: Think: If he does plan something, do you criticize his choice or decide you have a better plan? If this is the case and he doesn't seem to have a problem with it, then forget about it. You wouldn't be happy if he did start to make plans.

However, you should make sure that you aren't bossing him and others into a "my way or no way" situation. Wear the other shoes and ask your boyfriend and friends what they want to do. And make sure you don't ask just to say, "I have a better idea." While people generally do appreciate it if one person takes over most of the planning, they still like to feel their ideas are valued.

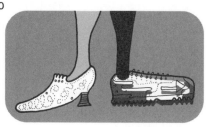

LAURA'S TIP: Guys are dopes. They usually think that everything will happen and they don't need to lift a finger. I have a guy friend who always says he has a great time hanging with me, but he has never once picked up the phone to make plans—it's always left up to me. It's not that he doesn't want to see me, but he just doesn't think of it.

I think their mothers do too much for them. I have lots of girlfriends with brothers who hardly have to help around the house at all. Your boyfriend probably doesn't even realize how lame he is. Tell him that you would really like to not have the responsibility of keeping the relationship together. He needs to take a part in it, too.

If you can't even count on him making a date, ask him if he's planning to spend next Friday night with you. Because if not, you're going to make other plans.

Jealousy

The cause for most jealousy is pretty simple: *fear.* Fear of getting dumped.

The trick is figuring out what's normal jealousy and what's not.

....

This girl at school is trying to steal my boyfriend. She hangs around him all the time. What am I supposed to do?

....

DR. MARLIN: Why is it that girls get angry with the girl instead of their cheating boyfriend? By blaming the other girl, you're thinking that your boyfriend still adores you—he's just such a fabulous catch that everyone wants him. But it usually takes two people to carry on a flirtation.

A boyfriend isn't a possession. No one can "steal" him without his permission.

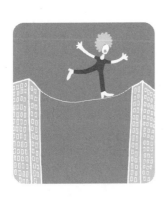

Talk to him and ask him what he wants. This is taking a risk. He may say he wants the other girl. In which case, of course, you are better off without him. But that doesn't mean you'll feel any better about being rejected. It hurts when someone does not want to go out with you anymore.

But this is going to happen as you start dating more. It doesn't mean you are a loser. Take it in stride that not every person you're attracted to is going to respond in the same way.

LAURA: Are you sure you're not just being overly jealous? A girl in my soccer league is convinced that every girl is after her boyfriend. She tells us all, "Hands off"—as if we'd want him in the first place.

But if you are just worried about this one girl, then don't do anything. If you say something to her, she'll only think she's making headway. If your boyfriend says something, she'll feel rejected and stop.

DR. MARLIN'S TIP: At the root of jealousy there is usually a feeling of being abandoned or unloved. Children of divorce, for example, are all too familiar with what it feels like for a loved one to depart suddenly. They may fear that abandonment will happen to them again. As a result, they may protect themselves in ways that are obsessive and controlling.

Studies show that while neither gender is more jealous than the other, jealousy is triggered by different factors in males and females. Female jealousy regularly revolves around the loss of emotional commitment from a partner—for example, e-mailing another girl. Male jealousy focuses more often on a partner's sexual infidelity.

Jealousy does have a productive side. Sometimes it can remind of you of what you want or what you take for granted. For instance, you may not have been sure about your relationship until you realized that someone else was also interested in your boyfriend.

But for the most part, it just eats a hole in your stomach, which then burns a hole in your confidence. Try to rearrange your thinking. Here's how:

1. Remember that the world is full of trustworthy guys with whom you can find happiness.
2. This is one time you should not talk about your feelings. No one wants to constantly have to prove his love for you. For instance, don't tell him that you feel upset if he talks to a skinny woman at a party. His conversation isn't making you feel fat—you probably had doubts about how you looked before you went out.
3. Accept his friendships with other women. The next time you feel like you are becoming gripped with jealousy, use this quick reality check. Ask yourself these questions:
   • Does she know about you?
   • Does he tell her good things or bad things about your relationship?
   • Does he talk to you about her all the time?

If you answered no, bad, and yes, then there's a soundness to your jealousy. He is not making you a priority in his life.

My boyfriend had sex with another girl. He says he's sorry and it won't happen again. Should I take him back?

DR. MARLIN: This is a very personal decision that's really about trust. Trust is important: If you can't rely on a guy to do what he says he'll do, be where he says he'll be, and carry through on promises, the relationship can't go forward or even stand still.

The fact that he's come clean shows there's hope for him. Does he seem really sorry? One way to tell is how he apologizes. "I'm sorry" are two of the easiest words to say. He should also have a sense that he really appreciates how hurt you are. For instance, is he taking full responsibility for his actions? The fact that you were away for the summer (and thus shifting the blame on you), he's a guy, he got seduced, he got drunk—none of these are excusable and none of them say, "I was wrong. It was me who made this mistake and hurt you. This has nothing to do with your behavior."

Also, can you begin to trust him again? Trust involves more than letting your boyfriend see you minus mascara. Trusting a guy means that you're sure he'll stick with you during the tough times, not just when you're having fun.

If you really want to know how he truly feels, look at his actions: He gives up a weekend to help you prepare for a big test; he cheers rather than sulks when you beat him at handball. Even the words "I love you" don't count. "Listen" to his actions.

Lastly, is your coupleship generally strong? Sex is the sharing of the body parts. It lasts about half an hour. Love is the feeling that the two of you share almost everything. It lasts much longer.

If the answer to these questions is yes, then it's probably fairly safe to forgive him. But there are no guarantees. Studies show that a person who cheats once is likely to cheat again.

LAURA: He shared the most intimate thing two people can share with someone other than you. As far as I'm concerned, he doesn't deserve to be forgiven. Do you really need someone you love to tell you (by his actions) that you are not the most desirable thing in the world to him?

Every girl I know whose boyfriend has cheated wastes good energy obsessing: Wasn't I good enough for him? What does she have that I don't? It's horrible. Their self-confidence has been shattered.

So I'm not even sure I would listen to him if he tried to apologize, because there is nothing he could say or do that would ever make me want to give him another chance.

Breaking Up

Every relationship is different. But most breakups are depressingly similar. No one can wave a wand and make the pain go away. No one can prove to you that you will love again. But it is within your power to take control of your breakup.

> My boyfriend and I just broke up. Even though it was something we both wanted, it's killing me whereas he seems totally fine. Why isn't he hurting like me?

DR. MARLIN: He probably *is* hurting, but in a different way. Research has found that women talk to say what they are feeling, but men tend express their emotions through action. For instance, if a guy loves you, rather than actually say the words, he might wash your car or fix your CD player. Conversely, if he is upset, he might take it out on the football field or go for a run.

But whether you're the leaver or the left, relationship breakup temporarily robs you of a sense of control over your life. Breaking up, regardless of whose idea it was, leads to some form of grief. You both will invariably go through different stages as you work through your pain (see Chapter 5):

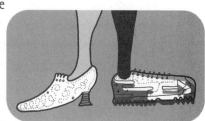

1. *Denial.* We're not over.
2. *Depression.* I will never find anyone like him/her again.
3. *Bargaining.* If I call you every night, can we still go out?
4. *Anger.* Fine, I don't want you either.
5. *Acceptance.* It's over.

The length of time it takes to get through each stage is individual. You might wallow in one stage and zip through another.

Watch out for the "I could have . . . I should have . . . I would have" statements. Many people fear that if someone rejects them, there must be something terribly wrong with them. The person who's getting dumped feels, "If only I had been more this or less that, he'd still want to be with me." This is putting the entire blame on your shoulders. Remember, a relationship is a two-way street.

Here's how to survive relationship breakup:

Fill your new free time wisely. Instead of wasting your time driving by his house 10 times a day to see if his car is there, make a list of his habits. You'll see that he wasn't such a perfect boyfriend after all. Then ask yourself how you want to be treated, what you deserve in a relationship, and if you got it from your ex. The answer is probably not.

Stop wallowing. Instead, try the following, even if you don't feel like it (fake it if you have to): Throw yourself into your schoolwork, read a book, take up a new sport—anything that will get you out there doing something to keep your mind off your ex. Friends can also help out by talking these feelings through with you.

Cry and scream. Just sob and let it all out. Many people ignore or deny the pain they're feeling. They pretend they're fine, that the relationship didn't mean that much to them. But if you don't let yourself feel everything that accompanies a breakup now, those feelings are just going to drag on and wear and tear you up from the inside out.

Talk it out. Go ahead and use your friends and family to unload.

Reprogram. Stop mid-sentence if you've been obsessing about what you could have–should have–would have done differently. Instead, change your chant to what you can't–won't–shouldn't ever do in a relationship again.

Reorganize. Stash or trash everything that reminds you of your ex. Sign up for kickboxing classes on a day that used to be your time together. Instead of lying around sobbing over him, pretend you're smashing him to pieces.

Put your pain in perspective. Watch the world news. Listen to country music. Watch a daytime talk show. Throw an ex party. Only those who have recently broken up can come.

Exercise your heart. A brisk walk, a run, or any aerobic activity will give you an endorphin rush—feel-good, all-natural chemicals that not only kill your pain but also make you feel strong and self-confident.

Start a journal. Or, if you already have one, write in it. You can also write your ex a letter telling him how much he is losing out on life without you and also (possibly) how much you miss him and want to hug him one last time. Then rip it up (you will regret it if you actually send it).

Get outside help. If a month passes and you still can't study, see your friends, get along with your parents, and/or you are eating/drinking too much or too little, then you're stalled in your grief and may need to talk to a professional to get moving (see Chapter 5).

This may seem like small stuff, but it's only when you start dealing that you'll feel back in the groove and be able to move on. In other words, regain your independence. A rich life will make the breakup less crushing, if only by distracting you from its sting.

Above all, don't conclude that love isn't worth it. Your broken relationship was not a waste of time. Through breakups you become more prepared to deal with future disappointments of all kinds—not just with guys.

They also teach you how to protect yourself from pain down the road by showing you what you want and don't want from relationships. Namely, you want a boyfriend who values you.

....

Two months after I dumped my boyfriend, another girl in my group started seeing him. I thought I was over him, but I'm really confused. Does this mean I still love my ex?

....

DR. MARLIN: It's normal to have mixed feelings when you see another girl on your ex's arm, especially when it's your close friend. Memories come rushing back and maybe you even wonder if you made a mistake.

But your jealousy is caused by one or a combination of these things:

1. *Rivalry with your friend.* He may seem to prefer her to you and/or have told her a thing or two about you that you'd rather she didn't hear—or vice versa (see Chapter 6).

2. *Latent possessiveness of your ex's life.* This is more complicated. It's only human to think that because you were there first he should love you best, and all future girlfriends should pale in comparison. But he can't very well sit in a room ticking off the hours until you come back.

3. *Insecurity.* You may think he is trading up with her. You need to shift your focus off of them and back to yourself. What they do or don't do has nothing to do with you. Remember, people are pretty much self-involved—their relationship is most likely about *them,* not about you.

4. *Still wanting him.* Sometimes we really don't know what we want until we lose it. If this is the case, it's something you have to work out with him, not with her. But think it through before you do or say anything. Are you just being territorial? Be careful—you may end up with a guy you don't want and without a friend you do.

LAURA: I can't even see a friend wear an old pair of shoes I've given her without wanting them back. I think it's hard making decisions about love and easy to think you are making the wrong one. When I see an old boyfriend, I always wonder what could have been and forget what was.

But you broke up with him for a reason. That reason has not disappeared. Remind yourself of it daily until your feelings of wanting him back go away.

Here's how to deal when you run into him:

First postbreakup encounter. Accept that you're probably going to hate how you look, even if you look fantastic. Keep things short and sweet. Nod and say, "Hey," and keep on walking to a friend with whom you can cry, get angry, yell, and moan.

Seeing him talking with another girl. Resist the urge to assume he's flirting. Instead, give him a small smile, nod, and walk on—don't run—straight to a friend . . . you know the drill.

Arranging to return each other's stuff. Get a friend to do it for you. Or arrange a blind drop-off in front of each other's house. You're probably already seeing each other every day at school. Why torture yourself more?

Meeting at a party and "accidentally" getting together. It happens—a lot. So don't dwell or assume that this means you are together again. If you want to clear the air, call him and tell him how you feel (for example, you miss him, if that's the case; it was a one-time thing, if that's the case). If he doesn't want to talk about it, think of it as your good-bye kiss.

Bumping into him and his new girlfriend. Smile. Ask how he's doing. Say hi to the new girl. This will show him that you're not bothered by his new relationship and it will make you feel strong. Then find the nearest friend. Unless you're with your new boyfriend. In which case, don't start telling all the gory moments of your breakup. If your new boyfriend asks about the other guy, just say, "We used to go out."

Quiz: Ex Love

You miss him. You're miserable. But before you try to get your ex back, think about which of the following best describes your current reality:

  a) "I can see where things went wrong in our relationship and how we can work it out this time."
  b) "Getting back together with my ex is better than being miserable and alone."
  c) "I plan to dump his sorry ass the minute he takes me back so that he can see how it feels."

Scoring

It's (a) or nothing. Any other answer means that you're still hurting and it's not a good idea to try to get back together and risk the pain when you're already down.

One Last Love Tip from Dr. Marlin

Quiz: Do You Really Want Him Back?

Answer the following to see if your relationship has staying power:

❑ *Does he tickle you?* It's not enough to have a sense of humor. You also need to get to each other's funny side.

❑ *Do you like him the way he is?* If you're thinking, "He's all right, but with a few tweaks to his hair, clothes, accent, personality, . . . he'll be perfect," stop right now. Boyfriends aren't works in progress and justifiably resent it if you criticize their taste (even if they don't have any).

❑ *Can he play Double Jeopardy with you?* If you feel he's intellectually challenged compared to you, you're going to be bored, no matter how cute he is.

❑ *Does he make you feel good?* You don't want him to make you the center of his universe (think smothered), but he should at least make you feel like his brightest star.

❑ *Does just looking at him make you melt?* When you meet a new guy, your brain pumps out hormones that tell you whether to go for it. There has to be some heat between you. How to tell? When you're magnetically drawn, your heart flips even though no one else has a clue as to what you see in him.

Scoring

If you checked at least four: You have the makings of a strong relationship. You connect, you respect each other, and you care about what's important to each other.

If you checked fewer than four: Looks like you two are more than casual acquaintances, but you're not quite soul mates. But don't give up hope—you may just be a pair in progress. The most important thing is that there's more than just lust between you. If, however, after 3 months you're still checking fewer than four boxes, the two of you would probably make better friends than a romantic couple.

3
Getting Physical

Dealing with your sexuality is confusing. Surveys show boys feel pressure to lose their virginity and girls feel pressure to keep it. Meanwhile, you're dealing with boyfriends who want sex, girlfriends who are having sex, and music and movies that send the message that sex will make you feel attractive and happy. Parents or teachers may say you're too young but talk to you as if you are sexually active.

Think of this chapter as an encyclopedia for finding out about sex and sexuality. It answers all the questions that you may not be able to ask your parents and has information that your friends may not know.

First Base

··

I've never kissed a guy and I'm scared I won't know how to do it.

··

DR. MARLIN: Let's get this out of the way: There is no right or wrong way. You just meet his lips and do whatever feels natural. But it does help to mellow out (which is hard, I admit, when you're nervous). The best kisses happen when you're relaxed. When you are comfortable mentally, your body will feel comfortable, which in turn will relax the muscles in your mouth and lips and make the kiss sweeter.

First kisses are nerve-racking for a boy, too, so don't think that he is going to be judging you. He may worry that you will think he doesn't know what he is doing.

Don't rush it—a slow kiss is far sexier than a quick and hard one. And it will give you time to feel comfortable putting your lips against his.

LAURA'S TIP: Try practicing. Imagine your mouth is like a goldfish's (don't laugh—this works) and then make those blow-out movements. That's all there is to it. Honest. Except for remembering to breathe!

Before my first time, I was so freaked, and then it turned out to feel so natural and easy that I don't know what I was worried about—it was like my lips knew what to do.

One girl I know was so uptight that she missed the guy's mouth and ended up licking his cheek! But they laughed about it and she knew they would be a good couple because they were comfortable together.

··

What's a French kiss?

··

DR. MARLIN: Any kissing that involves your tongue and his tongue touching.

DR. MARLIN'S TIP: It may feel strange at first, but it soon feels very nice. Start slow, with a soft lip kiss, then let your mouth open slightly and edge your tongue into his mouth until your tongues touch. The rest will come naturally.

....

I think about sex all the time. Is this normal?

....

DR. MARLIN: Yes. (But it's also normal not to think about sex all the time.) Your hormones are on high and everything can make you feel sexy—romantic movies, being with your boyfriend or even thinking about him, riding your bike, the sun on your shoulders, whatever! Thinking about sex can be a good way to mentally check out experiences.

LAURA: Boys and girls and sex and dating and hooking up are what we talk about most of the time. So it'd be weird if you didn't think about it a lot. Guys do and they don't worry, so why should we?

Second Base

....

My boyfriend touched my breasts and I didn't feel anything. Is that strange?

....

DR. MARLIN: Not at all. Maybe you were too nervous to relax and enjoy the feeling. Then there's the trust factor—what works when you're by yourself or with a longtime boyfriend may not work with a guy who is pressuring you to do something you're not ready for. Or this kind of stimulation may not be a turn-on for you. There is no rule that says all girls love having their breasts touched. Some love it, some think it's nice, and others don't feel much at all.

Sexual pleasure depends on more than stimulation: your mood, your feelings about your partner, even where you are in your menstrual cycle. Some women's breasts get very tender before their period and can't tolerate any touching. Keep your mind open and let your boyfriend know how you feel about what he is doing—or, for that matter, not doing.

Third Base

Two Views of the Female Sex Organs

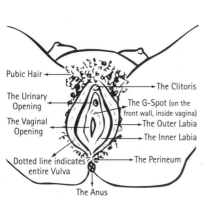

External Sex Organs
(also called genitals)

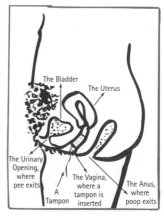

Internal Sex Organs
(side view)

Two Views of the Male Sex Organs

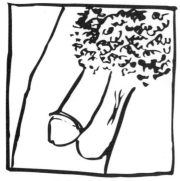

A flaccid penis

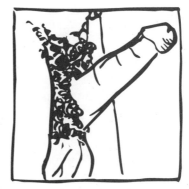

An erect penis

What is oral sex?

DR. MARLIN: Oral sex is when you put your mouth, lips, or tongue on a guy's penis (also known as fellatio), or he puts his mouth on your geni-

The Basics of Oral Sex

Your step-by-step guide for fellatio (blow job, giving/getting head, sucking off, gobbing the knob, giving/getting a hummer, sucking the root):

1. Suck or lick the penis while stroking its base with your hand.
2. Don't try to fit it all into your mouth, because you probably can't without tickling the back of the throat, which can make you gag.
3. Your boyfriend can show you how he likes to be stroked with his own hand and can tell you when he likes what you're doing (don't be embarrassed—be happy he's comfortable showing you what turns him on).
4. The key is to cover your teeth with your lips as much as possible and use lots of pressure. Make sure you don't

tal area, for example, your clitoris (also known as cunnilingus). When two people give each other oral sex at the same time, it is called "69."

You can't get pregnant from swallowing sperm, only by sperm entering your vagina. However, you can get STDs (sexually transmitted diseases) from oral sex. Nearly any disease you can get from intercourse you can also get from oral sex, and some STDs, such as herpes, are easier to catch orally (see "Love Sick" on page 85).

My boyfriend wants me to give him oral sex, but it sounds gross. Am I weird or is he?

DR. MARLIN: Neither of you is. Oral sex is like cuddling or kissing—it can be fabulous if you're both into it and unappetizing—even disgusting—if you're not. While you may think putting your mouth on his penis is revolting, it can be heaven for him. And lots of women enjoy it.

bite or scrape with your teeth, or rub the penis with a dry hand—neither is pleasurable for most men.

Your step-by-step guide for showing him how to give you cunnilingus (eating out, going down on, carpet munching, rug munching, chow box, muff diving):

1. Oral sex for women involves licking and sucking the vulval area.
2. You want your partner to give the most attention to the clitoris and the area around it, including the outer and inner labia (vaginal lips), the vaginal opening, and the perineum (the bit of flesh between your anal hole and vaginal opening).
3. Let him know what you like and don't like by moaning or telling him when something feels good. Nothing is as important as voicing your likes and dislikes.

LAURA: If you're curious about it, then you may want to. But if you think giving some guy a blow job will make you popular or he'll like you, then you only want what comes along with doing it. In that case, I wouldn't, because it wouldn't be for me and my pleasure.

DR. MARLIN'S TIP: If you give it a try, use a condom. Oral sex is in the risk category for HIV (human immunodeficiency virus), syphilis, genital herpes, HPV (human papilloma virus or genital warts), gonorrhea, and chlamydia.

Flavored condoms make this safer as well as tastier—they come in cherry, strawberry, chocolate, to name a few.

61

•••

This guy and I were kissing when his pants suddenly got all wet. He pretended nothing happened. Did he pee in his pants?

•••

DR. MARLIN: Actually, he lost control and ejaculated. The liquid was semen, which is made up of milky fluids and sperm. Involuntary ejaculation happens when guys first start getting sexual because their penises are very responsive to stimulus.

Your boyfriend was probably mortified. How you handle this is a mark of how good a girlfriend you are. You could be embarrassed and act awkward. But think, "My period stained through my white jeans" and you'll get a sense of what he's feeling. You'd be embarrassed and hope your friends would be sympathetic, help you clean up, and get on with normal conversation ASAP. Same thing applies here.

DR. MARLIN'S TIP: If he ejaculated near your genitals (your vagina and behind) or on your hands and you then touched your genitals, go to a gynecologist to be checked out for pregnancy and STDs.

Home Base

Quiz: Are You Ready to Get Intimate?

1. A guy you like asks you out to an expensive dinner. When it comes time to say good-night, you:
   a) Say, "Thanks, I had a great time."
   b) Give him a kiss on the cheek.
   c) Fool around a little. After all, he did spend all that money on you.

2. You're ready for sex. You:
   a) Get latex condoms and spermicide.
   b) Skip the protection. You don't need to worry the first time.
   c) Leave it up to your boyfriend.

3. You need to borrow your guy's car for a true emergency. You:
   a) Think about asking him, but decide not to. You know he'll never lend it no matter what.
   b) Figure you'll call him if no one else can help you.
   c) Call him right away. You know he loves you enough to trust you won't crash it.

4. You had sex and now you've missed your period. Would you tell your boyfriend?
   a) Absolutely. You're going to need his help and support.
   b) Maybe. What if he freaks?
   c) No way. He'd probably dump you flat-out.

5. You're fooling around with your boyfriend when things start getting too hot to handle. He tells you he's too excited to stop and he loves you. You:
   a) Go ahead and do it. You don't want to ruin your relationship.
   b) Ditch him on the spot.
   c) Firmly tell him to calm down, saying, "I like being with you, but I'm just not ready."

6. Who would you ask about birth control?
   a) Your friends.
   b) No one.
   c) Your folks or some other adult you trust.

Answers

1.	a. 3	b. 2	c. 1
2.	a. 3	b. 1	c. 2
3.	a. 1	b. 2	c. 3
4.	a. 3	b. 2	c. 1
5.	a. 1	b. 2	c. 3
6.	a. 2	b. 1	c. 3

Scoring

6–10: JUST SAY NO.

No way are you ready. If you're already having sex, *stop!* You should be in control, which means that you can always stop or not do it again, even if you've already done it once.

First, read this chapter (especially the questions on birth control and what to do if a guy pressures you) and Chapter 2 (especially about trust) over again.

Next, talk to him. If you're uncomfortable talking about it, you're not ready to do it.

Lastly, ask yourself why you want to have sex, why you want to have sex with *him,* why he wants to have sex with *you,* and why now. Then take this quiz again and see how you score. Better to be certain than sorry.

11–15: ALMOST THERE.

In many ways, you know how to take care of yourself and have a fairly honest relationship. But you're not 100 percent sure that you're ready to go all the way.

In that case, don't. Sex should be what you'll feel good about before, during, and afterward. Having it too soon, without protection, or with the wrong guy is not going to leave you happy or even sexually satisfied. So wait—at least until you nudge your score over 14.

Here are the worst reasons to have sex (and that includes letting him feel you up and having oral sex):

✳ To be cool
✳ To be with the in crowd
✳ To get boyfriends

Here are the best reasons to have sex:

✳ You love each other.
✳ You've talked about it and how you will feel about it.
✳ You've shared plans about birth control.
✳ It feels like a natural progression of your relationship (not something forced or so weird you feel sick about it).

16–18: YOU'RE READY.

You've got knowledge and confidence. You're not using sex to keep your boyfriend interested, you're prepared on the protection front, and you trust your guy to love you and be there for you no matter what. This doesn't mean you *have* to have sex. Being ready also means knowing when it's better not to—being willing to wait until the timing and situation are totally right.

....

What exactly happens during sex?

....

DR. MARLIN: First, you get aroused by kissing and necking (also known as first base). Second, you touch and kiss each other everywhere above the waist (second base). Third, petting progresses with you touching and kissing each other's genitals (third base).

This foreplay can last as long as you want. He'll get an erection (and should put on a condom), and you will feel very hot and tense, but in a good way. You may feel wetness in your groin. This is known as lubrication, which your body produces to ease penetration (his inserting his penis into your vagina).

These first three steps are also the first two stages of orgasm (there are four altogether). In the first stage, *arousal/excitement,* blood rushes to the genitals, causing engorgement. Erection in the male and vaginal lubrication in the female are visible signs.

After rapidly climbing excitement, there is a leveling off of sexual tension, which is known as the *plateau.* This can last as long as you want.

The third stage involves a pleasurable release of sexual tension, known as *orgasm.* In men, it involves ejaculation. As he gets closer to orgasm and ejaculation, his thrusts will get faster. Most women need clitoral stimulation to reach orgasm and often require a longer period of stimulation. Given the differences, most couples do not have simultaneous orgasms.

In the final phase, known as *resolution,* the body gradually returns to a quiet state. Men need time before getting another erection (perhaps 15 minutes for teenage boys, an hour or more for older men). Women are capable of multiple orgasms (as long as they are being stimulated).

Unimaginably strong emotions accompany these stages. At the height of physical passion, people feel they have never been so in love, so con-

Getting
Physical

nected, that they can't live without their lover, they belong to their lover, they'd do anything for their lover. They say things they might not say at any other time (for example, "I love you") and mean it—at the moment.

DR. MARLIN'S TIP: Some things can interfere with lubrication. The pill affects all parts of the body with synthetic hormones, which can cause changes that result in vaginal dryness. Nervous tension and fatigue may contribute to this problem as well.

K-Y Jelly or Lubafax are lubricants placed directly into the vagina to provide quick lubrication. Astroglide simulates lubrication for a longer period of time. Lubrin inserts are premeasured to simulate the body's natural lubrication for several hours and may be inserted 5 to 30 minutes before intercourse.

....
What does an orgasm feel like?
....

DR. MARLIN: No two are alike. First, there are physical changes: The skin flushes, the tissues fill with blood, and the breasts enlarge. As arousal moves to orgasm, there are spiking blood pressure and pulse, as well as anal and vaginal contractions. The main event—supreme pleasure followed by a feeling of well-being and satiation—occurs in the brain's limbic system or pleasure center. The buildup can last minutes or even hours, but the female orgasm is about 19 to 28 seconds long, with an average of 23 (the male climax lasts only a few seconds).

Orgasm can vary, depending on level of arousal and type of stimulation (masturbation, intercourse, oral sex, clitoral touching) to achieve it, and your mood and physical well-being. It can range from mild pleasure to being so overwhelming that you momentarily lose consciousness. It may be intense or relaxing. You might feel a ripple of warmth through your body or almost a tickle. Sometimes, you may feel disoriented or dizzy.

Most orgasms result from stimulating the clitoris, but they can vary. There is "blended" orgasm, in which vaginal stimulation contributes as well. The elusive G-spot is an area on the front wall of your vagina, inside the vaginal walls. Some women enjoy G-spot stimulation and some don't. Some women experience multiple orgasms—that is, a series of orgasms following one another. Others do not. Most women first experience orgasm through masturbation (see "Solo Sex" on page 75) rather than intercourse.

Some women don't know when they've had an orgasm, or don't trust in it, because a lot of myths have confused the matter. Though it is a marvelous feeling, you may not always scream, the earth doesn't always move, nor does your head feel as if it were being blown off. The best way to know you've had one is if you feel satisfied.

DR. MARLIN'S TIP: Reaching orgasm is wonderful, and in time you'll learn how to have one, but it's a bit like eating dinner: The point isn't to finish what's on your plate and rush away from the table. Just as you should savor each bite, you should relish giving your body what it wants and needs, at its own pace.

Mellow out. There's a very strong brain–body link between relaxing and orgasm. The more pressured, unsure, uptight, or scared you feel, the less your body can do what it needs to do.

First, you have to be aroused, feel sexual energy, ready to go ahead, which in turn gets your nerve endings tingling, your blood flowing, and your body producing vaginal lubrication. Then, as sexual tension builds, you feel as if your entire body were clenched, ready to explode. When orgasm comes, it's an incredible release of all the built-up tension. That's the physical part.

The mental part is that you let go completely and feel utterly and completely vulnerable, close, and open with your partner. To enjoy sex, you have to be comfortable in your body and with your partner, and be sure that you've taken adequate precautions (you can't let go if you're worried about getting pregnant or getting an STD).

Nine Orgasmic Truths for Women

1 About 60 percent of all women discovered orgasm alone (typically through masturbation).

2 Around 23 percent had their first orgasm by age 15.

3 Approximately 40 percent have had nocturnal orgasms (similar to men's wet dreams).

4 About 70 percent have masturbated to orgasm.

5 About 26 percent of women ages 18 to 35 have used a vibrator to orgasm.

6 Around 30 percent reach orgasm through intercourse.

7 About 75 percent require clitoral stimulation to orgasm.

8 Up to 66 percent have faked an orgasm.

9 Approximately 10 percent have never had an orgasm.

Some women fake orgasm, feeling they are disappointing their partner if they don't come. This is a bad habit because it gives your partner false cues about what turns you on.

....

How will I know when I'm ready to go all the way?

....

DR. MARLIN: Do these five basic conditions apply? (1) You're with someone you trust. (2) You've talked about sex and birth control and about what happens if you get pregnant. (3) You don't feel pressured to do something you don't want to do. (4) You're nervous (it goes with the territory), but you don't feel like the future of your relationship is at stake. (5) You're listening to your heart as well as your head.

Although 56 percent of women and 73 percent of men today have intercourse by age 18, that doesn't mean they are happy about it. A recent study found that both guys and girls who waited until they were 17 or older enjoyed the experience much more than those who had intercourse earlier.

LAURA: You should be happy and excited more than scared or worried about if it will hurt or if you really want to do it. Ask yourself how you'd feel if you two broke up the next day. I know if I kiss somebody and he doesn't call afterward, it's terrible. And that's such a smaller deal than sex.

....

My boyfriend keeps pressuring me, but I'm not ready.

....

DR. MARLIN: Then shout it out. Keeping quiet will only hurt you and your relationship. So tell him. If he can't respect your feelings and wishes, then he's not right for you.

If he says:	You should say:
You'd do it if you loved me.	You wouldn't pressure me if you loved me.
Everyone else is doing it.	Then do it with them.
You're a tease.	You're selfish and inconsiderate.
You're immature.	I know what I want—and right now it's *not* you, babe.
It's not good for me to get all excited and not have any release.	Then go masturbate.

Just in case you think there's no way he can control himself, know that recent polls show that when 10,000 teenagers—guys and girls—were

Laura's Top 10 Excellent Reasons Not to Have Sex

10 You don't want to and that's all there is to it.

9 You think it'll make you popular.

8 He says you'd do it if you really loved him.

7 You think you'll never see him again unless . . .

6 You barely know him.

5 You haven't even talked about protection.

4 You're scared.

3 All your friends are doing it.

2 You think you'll die from frustration if you don't.

1 You don't know how to say no.

asked the question, "Can sexual urges be controlled?" 51 percent said "Always"; just 3.5 percent said "Never."

••

My boyfriend knows I've had sex before and assumes that I'll sleep with him, but I don't want to.

••

DR. MARLIN: Because you did something once, twice, or even a hundred times does not mean you have to keep doing it. The point of making love is that it be mutually fun, cozy, and comfortable—definitely not something you are pushed or rushed into doing.

Getting Physical

Dr. Marlin's Simple No-Thanks-to-Sex Action Plan

1. Make the decision to stay true to your ideals (you may have moral or religious reasons not to have sex). Write down your own personal limits (you will kiss, but you won't let him touch your breasts; you can finger each other, but no oral sex, etc.).

2. Be up front with guys you date. Make sure they understand and respect your decision. Do it without sounding defensive or like you're challenging them to try something. Timing is also important. Bring it up too soon and it sounds like you're pushing the relationship. Wait too long and it's just uncomfortable. Keep it short and sweet and matter of fact as if you expect him to agree. If he gives you any trouble and keeps trying to convince you you're wrong, decide you are wrong—for each other.

3. Think about where you want to be, say, 5 years from now. That goal probably does not include being a mom or being sick with an STD.

DR. MARLIN'S TIP: Anyone who tries to make you do what is uncomfortable is not a guy you want to be with. You will have sexual feelings, but you can choose to act on them or not. If you decide to have sex responsibly and safely and feel good about it, that doesn't make you a slut. If you feel best being abstinent, you're not a prude.

But that decision has to come from you—not current or potential partners, or family or friends. *Your sexuality is yours.*

I want to have sex, but my boyfriend doesn't want to. What's wrong with him?

DR. MARLIN: Nothing. Some boys aren't ready but think that if they're "real" guys they should be pressuring you. Your guy seems to know he's not ready. That makes him smart and courageous, willing to be himself. So try seeing things from his side. Respect what he wants—as you'd want to be respected if you were the one who wanted to wait.

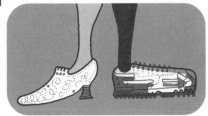

DR. MARLIN'S TIP: Sex is like hiking with someone: Always go at the slower person's pace. It can lead to wonderful explorations along the way.

My boyfriend and I tried to have sex, but he couldn't get it in. What's wrong?

DR. MARLIN: Tension, tightness, nerves, and shoving instead of gently maneuvering can make penetration difficult. Or he may be trying to stick it in the wrong place. The more foreplay you have, the more your body produces lubrication and the easier penetration will be (see "What Exactly Happens During Sex?" on page 65 for more on lubrication). Insertion can also be difficult if he's not fully erect.

We went too far and I don't know how to keep
things in control next time.

DR. MARLIN: Have a plan. Knowing in advance what you want is the way to be sure you will make the right choice for you in the heat of the moment.

First, don't blame yourself for losing control. When something feels good, it's difficult to stop. But just because you did it once doesn't mean you have to do it again.

Once you decide what feels comfortable (he should be doing the same), sit down and set guidelines *before* you get physical again. Tell him how much you care for him but that you don't feel good going that far, and be clear on what you want to do from now on. He may even be relieved. Many boys feel they must pressure you to prove their masculinity, even if they are not ready for sex themselves.

Getting
Physical

DR. MARLIN'S TIP: If a physical encounter is getting out of control, it's never too late to slow down. Simply take his hand, gently remove it from where it's headed, and say, "I really like you, but I don't want to do this now." If you're too embarrassed or shy to say this, you're especially not ready to be intimate with him.

What is backdoor sex?

DR. MARLIN: Slang for anal sex—when a guy puts his penis in your anus (butt). There is no risk of pregnancy, but anal tissue, unlike vaginal tissue, can't lubricate itself and is prone to tearing. Anal sex is a high-risk activity for getting the AIDS (autoimmune deficiency syndrome) virus and other STDs (sexually transmitted diseases) (see "Love Sick" on page 85).

Sperm in your anus can't make you pregnant, but it might run out and come in contact with your vagina, which *can* make you pregnant. So you need to use a condom.

Since your anus is tighter and narrower than your vagina, take it very slow. If you want to experiment, try a gloved and lubricated finger first—do not use baby oil, which can erode the latex in condoms. Use a water-based lubricant like K-Y Jelly. If you don't like the way it feels, a penis is probably not going to feel good.

··

I had sex and didn't like it. Is something wrong with me?

··

DR. MARLIN: Absolutely not. Often sex is uncomfortable the first time. It takes experience to discover your body and figure out what feels good. You may just be nervous doing something new, your body can't relax, neither of you knows what turns you on and off, and things may happen too quickly.

You may not know each other well enough to feel relaxed in such an intimate way. Because you like to be aroused and enjoy physical intimacy doesn't automatically translate into liking or wanting intercourse. If the first time is awful, your body may be saying, "I'm not ready." Listen to it.

Also, the position is important. The two best for first intercourse are either with the man on top (missionary) or with the woman on top. Being on top makes it easier to control how deeply you are penetrated. Go slow. Start by putting the tip of his penis against your vaginal opening, then let your partner know how deep to go, how fast to move. Don't do anything that feels uncomfortable; pain tells your body what not to do.

It may only feel good to have him penetrate you an inch and move very slowly. On the other hand, it may feel fine to have him enter more deeply and move more rapidly. Tell him what feels good and what doesn't.

If it hurts, stop. Take a couple of minutes to let the penis be pressed against your opening, perhaps stimulating your clitoris a little, or to hug and kiss. When you're ready, try again. You may have to do this several times, and it should still be enjoyable and intimate. In fact, you may not want to be fully penetrated on the first try. That's just fine. There should be no hurry.

You may not have an orgasm the first time from the intercourse itself.

Most women don't. That doesn't mean anything is wrong. Even when you're more experienced, it is possible that intercourse won't bring you to climax by itself, but that other forms of sex, like oral sex or manual clitoral stimulation combined with intercourse, will. Only 30 percent of women say they have orgasms from intercourse alone.

First intercourse isn't easy for guys, either. He may be just as nervous, scared, or inexperienced as you are and may feel the same pressure to perform. A young man may also fear hurting his partner and may lose his erection once, several times, or even for good during a session. That is perfectly normal (see condom tips on pages 93–94). Give him as much patience and sensitivity as you want him to give you.

DR. MARLIN'S TIP: Meanwhile, try self-discovery. What is satisfying, safe, and comfortable for you? Masturbating by yourself can help you get to know your body. When you are ready to do it again, you'll know what makes you feel good (see "Solo Sex" below).

Getting
Physical

Solo Sex

According to studies, 30 percent of women masturbate at least weekly and 95 percent do it some time in their lives.

•••

Sometimes I like to touch myself between my legs. Can this hurt me?

•••

DR. MARLIN: Masturbation is not bad for you physically, sexually, or emotionally. In fact, it's good for you (even the American Medical Association says so). It's a way to reduce stress, to relax, to learn what turns you on, to keep you happy when you're not ready for sex with a guy, and even to relieve menstrual cramps and headaches. Plus it feels good and it's the safest sex there is.

10 Sexy Alternatives to Sex

What's the rush? Of the 10 most important things in a solid love connection, sex is number 9 (in case you haven't figured it out, number 1 is respect). So the best test of a relationship is to see what happens when you hold off. Here are some amazingly sexy alternative ways to connect:

1 Unleash some butterfly kisses.

2 Have him paint your toenails (probably first on his secret wish list).

3 Share a hot-fudge sundae with one spoon.

4 Sit back-to-back and deeply inhale, then exhale, and feel each other's heartbeats through your backbones.

··

Why do I always have an orgasm when I masturbate, but I never have one with my boyfriend?

··

DR. MARLIN: Simple. *You* know what you like. So show your boyfriend how to touch you the way you touch yourself. Just take his hand and put it where you put your own, then move it like you move your own. He'll get the idea.

5 Charge your bodies with static electricity by rubbing your feet on a rug and then kiss. Make sure your lips are the first body parts to touch and watch the sparks fly.

6 Croon your song. Belt it out in the car together or whisper it in each other's ears while you're slow dancing to it.

7 Memorize each other's faces with your fingertips (no cheating—keep your eyes closed).

8 Pop a few Hershey kisses in your mouth and give him the sweetest kiss ever.

9 Give each other a long, long hug.

10 Make kissing history—the longest kiss ever lasted 417 hours!

My mother caught me masturbating. I don't know what to say to her.

DR. MARLIN: If she's not talking about it, let it go. It's private—there's really nothing to discuss. She may be uncomfortable and want to pretend it never happened.

If she starts lecturing you, tune her out. Your mother may think masturbation is evil, or that it ruins you for a man, or some other misguided viewpoint she learned as a girl.

From now on, lock the door. Or use the bathroom if your bedroom door doesn't have a lock.

Masturbation ABCs

There's no right or wrong way. No normal or abnormal methods. Each woman is unique and has her own pattern. So one might briskly rub herself whereas another might use the water from the showerhead. Some like to slowly caress their whole body, whereas others go directly for the genitals. Some women lie on their stomach and others on their back or side. Very few report they like direct stimulation of the tip or glans of the clitoris. It's very sensitive, and direct stimulation can be irritating or actually painful.

We all have different sexual fantasies. Someone who one day is aroused by the image of a romantic gentle lover may the next day fantasize about being overpowered by force. Both are okay. They're your fantasies, not your actions, and to think is not to do. It's also perfectly normal not to fantasize.

LAURA'S TIP: I know how horrible it feels when my mother walks into my room without knocking when I'm not doing anything, so I can only imagine how horrible it would be if she caught me doing that.

I don't even want to connect my mother and sex in the same thought. One time when I was 7 and I asked my mom what her favorite activity was, she just blurted out, "sex." I was too freaked for words.

I appreciate my mother being open with me about sex, but sometimes I wish she were less so. It almost makes it harder for me, because if I make a mistake like not using condoms, I *really* should know better.

You and your mom need to talk about privacy—yours and hers. She shouldn't walk in on you without knocking first, even if she does pay the rent. You might ask how she would feel if you wandered in on her without knocking (I'm assuming you respect her privacy as much as you want her to respect yours).

Being Gay

For most people, realizing they're gay or bisexual doesn't happen overnight. Perhaps you have had crushes on people of the same sex, or felt your gender or sexual roles just aren't comfortable for you. While these feelings certainly don't mean you are gay or bisexual, they are clues that you might be.

If you feel attracted to those of the same sex, you may worry that you might be gay. You may be afraid to admit your feelings because you think you will be branded in some way, or because you fear being rejected by your friends, family, or community. There are probably others in your area who feel the same sense of disconnection because of their sexual orientation, but they don't know how to reach out. You could look for gay/bisexual groups on-line (see "Address Book" on page 260).

If you do manage to get close with someone, you have a new set of problems. How public do you get? Do you tell your parents? What about your friends?

It's up to you to define who you are. This section will give you some things to consider.

....

I'm attracted to my girlfriend. We've kissed and touched a little, and I really enjoyed it. Does this mean I'm gay?

....

DR. MARLIN: No, there may be many reasons you feel the way you do now and not all of them have to do with sex.

Your sexual urges are in overdrive because your hormone levels are changing. Result: You're more easily turned on, even by girls.

Many people get off on the general idea of sex, not necessarily on thoughts of a specific person. Your attraction may not even have to do with sex. There may be things about your friend you admire and enjoy, like the cool way she walks, or that she looks really good, and getting physical with her is a way of acting out these feelings. Or perhaps you're reacting to the closeness between you as friends.

When you're an adolescent, it's common to have close feelings for other girls and even act them out yet actually be straight (just like gay girls sometimes have feelings for guys).

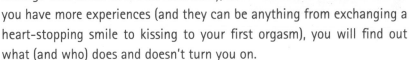

Part of sexual growth is riding it out and enjoying all the crazy, mixed-up feelings that come with sex. Eventually, as you have more experiences (and they can be anything from exchanging a heart-stopping smile to kissing to your first orgasm), you will find out what (and who) does and doesn't turn you on.

You don't have to decide right now whether you're straight or bisexual or gay. I don't know a heterosexual woman who hasn't had at least one romantic experience with women, especially in adolescent years. Whether it's unacted-on physical attraction, or a fantasy, or one hookup, it's normal, regardless of where you end up later.

LAURA: A girl from this club I was in had a crush on me. At first, I was repulsed—it just seemed too weird. Then I was intrigued. I couldn't imagine what two girls do together. Then she got a crush on a male friend of mine and I realized that it wasn't so much what I looked like that she was into but who I am. And that made me feel flattered. I still felt strange around her, but no more so than I would if she had been a guy who liked me who I wasn't interested in.

....

I'm Gay. Should I come out?

....

DR. MARLIN: Many people spend years of unhappiness denying their true feelings. Some take a long time to realize they're gay. So it's good you're so clear about it.

Coming out—letting the world know you're gay—is one of the hardest things you'll ever do. How family and friends react will depend on many factors, including their preconceived notions of what kind of life they envision for you, what they know about homosexuality (some people think it's a sin or sick), and how comfortable they are discussing such matters.

Are You Gay?

People who are gay can do just about everything sexually that people who are heterosexual do: kiss, have oral sex, touch each other's sexual organs, penetrate each other (lesbians may use a dildo, which is a penis-shaped tool).

There are certain clues that you may be gay or bisexual:

* Have you felt attracted to more than one or two members of the same sex?
* Do members of the same sex enter into your sexual fantasy life on a regular basis?
* Do you feel on some levels that you just don't fit in with others your age?
* Do you feel that typical gender roles (such as girls dressing up or being soft-spoken, or boys being into contact sports or acting gruff) don't fit you at all?
* Do you feel bored or just not excited going out with members of the other sex?
* Have you suspected you might be homosexual or bisexual?

Obviously, any of this can apply to heterosexuals as well as homosexuals, but if a few sound familiar, if you feel that way often, and you're at the stage of life where you are having a surge of hormones and some relationship experiences, you may be gay or bisexual.

No one but you can assign you an orientation or an identity. What you call yourself, how you identify, and when you identify (and this may not be solid—for some, it shifts) are your choices.

Getting Physical

81

Sometimes even people who love you react badly because they want what's best for you and don't believe that homosexuals can be happy. That's ridiculous.

Here's a short sampling from a long list of well-known people who are openly gay and happy: Ellen DeGeneres, Anne Heche, Rupert Everett, k. d. lang, Melissa Etheridge, George Michael, Elton John, Martina Navratilova, Congressman Barney Frank, and former Congressman Gerry Studds.

There is still hatred for homosexuals in our society, and those close to you may worry that you will be mistreated. A therapist colleague of mine couldn't accept his son's coming out—he was terrified his son would be ostracized—even though my colleague has counseled many gay clients who have had lots of wonderful friends and partners!

LAURA: Most gay people I know are out. I know they all feel better for not having to keep their sexuality a secret. But I also know the only rea-

Coming-Out Checklist

There are things you can do and say to make coming out easier:

* *To out or not to out.* Think about your relationships with people before coming out to them. Do you feel safe with them? How do you expect them to react? You don't want their responses to surprise you. There are many good sources for finding an ally to help you through this difficult process. See the "Address Book" on page 255 for people to call for specific advice.

* *Say the G-word.* Honesty is key. Tell as much as you can without being sexually graphic. You might simply say, "I'm gay," or relate it to a movie, TV show, or book: For example, "Remember the

son they don't get hassled is because they're fairly confident people in the first place.

But reactions can surprise you. I read about this popular captain of his school's football team who came out in his senior year after one of his uncles made a gay slur and his other uncle laughed. The whole team accepted it and supported him.

DR. MARLIN'S TIP: Questions to ask yourself when deciding whether to come out:

* Am I tired of secrecy and lying?
* Am I too lonely not sharing this with anyone?
* Do I have at least one good choice for who to tell first?
* Have I thought this through?
* Can I do it when I'm calm and there's time to talk in a private place?

character Rupert Everett played in *My Best Friend's Wedding?*" Be ready to answer questions. Because so many people are confused about homosexuality and bisexuality, explain what it means to you, and what is and isn't true for you.

* *Give them space.* Coming out might be a surprise, and even if your loved ones are fine with it, they may need time to adjust. Tell your parents in privacy so that they can gather their thoughts before they talk to others about it. And don't imagine their initial reaction indicates how they will finally feel.

* *Support them.* Give your family and friends access to books, Web sites, and organizations (see "Address Book" on page 260).

* *Don't apologize.* Never apologize for who you are.

Everything You Need to Know About STDs but Were Afraid to Ask

Quiz: Are You at Risk?

1. Are you female?
2. Are you under age 20?
3. Do you live in a city of more than 200,000?
4. Have you had sex with more than one partner in the past 3 months?
5. Have you had sex with a new partner in the past 3 months?
6. Are you too embarrassed to ask your partner about his sexual history?
7. Do you know or suspect your partner has had sex with others while he's been with you?
8. Have you ever had sex without using a condom?
9. Have you ever had sex with someone the first time you met?
10. Have you ever had an STD?
11. Have you ever had sex after using drugs or alcohol?
12. Have you or your partner ever used IV (intravenous) drugs?
13. Have you ever given someone money or drugs for sex?

Score

No "yes" answers: low risk

One to three "yes" answers: medium risk

Four or more "yes" answers: high risk—*always use a condom*

Love Sick

STDs don't disappear on their own. They must be treated.

AIDS (autoimmune deficiency syndrome)

WHAT: The end product of becoming infected with HIV (human immunodeficiency virus), a virus that attacks the immune system by infecting white blood cells. Eventually the infected person will not be able to fight off the illness and even the slightest cold will make her or him very sick, ultimately causing death. A person can carry HIV and not have signs of AIDS, although he or she will probably develop it.

HOW: HIV is spread through blood, semen, vaginal fluids, and breast milk.

SYMPTOMS: There may not be any for years, or shortly after infection the person may experience a flu-like illness, followed by a period of feeling good (but the person is still contagious). Other early symptoms include extreme fatigue, fever, weight loss, diarrhea, and night sweats.

PROTECTION: Avoid exchanging body fluids—blood, semen, vaginal fluids—with anyone you suspect is infected. Unprotected anal intercourse is the highest risk factor, followed closely by unprotected vaginal intercourse; oral sex is a much lower risk factor and saliva is the least risk. And women are much more vulnerable than men. Using a latex condom during intercourse and fellatio will greatly reduce risk.

When is it safe to stop using condoms in a relationship? Most gynecologists say if you've been mutually monogamous for 6 months, have both tested HIV negative, waited 6 months, and been retested with a negative result, then it's probably okay—but the sad truth is you may never know with certainty that your guy is trustworthy.

TIMING: AIDS can take from 6 months to 10 years to develop. A person will test HIV positive during this time, but may have no symptoms.

IF UNTREATED: Death.

TREATMENT: Early detection with a blood test and new drugs may prolong life. But there's no known cure.

Getting Physical

CHLAMYDIA

(cla-MIH-dee-ah)

WHAT: Bacterial infection of the genitals. The fastest-spreading STD out there, it affects about 4 million people a year, and it's more common among teens than older men and women—up to 29 percent of sexually active teenage girls and 10 percent of sexually active teenage boys have been found to have chlamydia.

HOW: Having vaginal, anal, or oral sex without a condom.

SYMPTOMS: A milky yellow vaginal discharge, genital itching/burning, dull stomach pain, and pain during peeing. But up to 75 percent of those infected have no symptoms at all.

PROTECTION: Only condoms offer protection, but they aren't 100 percent effective.

TIMING: 1 to 3 weeks after infection.

IF UNTREATED: Infertility, abnormal Pap smears, PID (pelvic inflammatory disease), or cervical infections.

TREATMENT: A 5-day course of antibiotics cures it. Both you *and* your partner need treatment before resuming sex. Otherwise, it'll leapfrog back and forth between you.

GENITAL WARTS

WHAT: Also known as HPV (human papillomavirus), this is a viral infection of the genital area or rectum.

HOW: Having unprotected vaginal, oral, or anal sex or touching a partner's infected area.

SYMPTOMS: *Highly contagious,* with painless smooth and/or cauliflower-like warts around genitals and anus.

PROTECTION: Condoms, though not 100 percent effective.

TIMING: 3 weeks to 8 months after contact.

IF UNTREATED: Some women with warts are at higher risk for gynecological problems like pelvic cramping, infertility, and cervical cancer. Some men are at higher risk for penile cancer.

TREATMENT: Painting the wart(s) with podophyllin or acetic acid, surgical removal with lasers, or cutting them out. But warts can come back. Regular examinations with Pap smears are the best bet for detection.

GONORRHEA ("THE CLAP")

(gone-o-RHEE-a)

WHAT: A bacterial infection.

HOW: Having unprotected vaginal, oral, or anal sex.

SYMPTOMS: If symptoms show up at all, a painful burning sensation during peeing and greenish vaginal discharge.

PROTECTION: It's highly contagious. Condoms provide the best barrier, although diaphragms and cervical caps used with spermicide are also effective.

TIMING: 80 percent of women and 10 percent of men with gonorrhea show no symptoms. If symptoms appear, they are present in women within 10 days. It takes 1 to 14 days for symptoms to appear in men.

IF UNTREATED: Infertility, arthritis, heart problems, and pelvic inflammatory disease.

TREATMENT: Antibiotics cure gonorrhea. Both partners must be treated, even if one doesn't have symptoms. You must avoid all sexual contact until cured.

HEPATITIS B

WHAT: One of five kinds of hepatitis viruses (A through E) that cause inflammation of the liver.

HOW: Having unprotected vaginal, oral, or anal sex.

SYMPTOMS: Many people have no symptoms or confuse their symptoms with flu: low fever, muscle aches, fatigue, loss of appetite, vomiting and diarrhea. Later, urine may be very dark, bowel movements may be pale, and eyes and skin have a yellowish (jaundice) tint.

PROTECTION: Condoms, though not 100 percent effective.

TIMING: Blood tests can detect the virus and antibodies.

IF UNTREATED: Cirrhosis of the liver, cancer of the liver.

TREATMENT: The only STD for which there is a vaccine.

HERPES

(her-PEAS)

WHAT: Many different types, but two main strains: HSV-1, which generally causes sores in the mouth area and is very common; and

HSV-2, which mainly causes sores in the genital area. But HSV-1 can appear genitally and HSV-2 can appear in the mouth and face region. Confusing, huh? Researchers guess as many as two-thirds of people with HSV-2 don't know they have it!

HOW: Rubbing and touching the infected area. The first attack is often the most contagious and painful.

SYMPTOMS: Itching, followed by painful blisters that rupture and become tender sores, which may make peeing painful. Sometimes symptoms don't pop up until years after you're infected, which is why you need to get tested by a doctor if you suspect you may have been infected. If symptoms appear, they may fade without treatment, but the sores can reoccur unpredictably, often when you're under stress or you have your period.

PROTECTION: In a single act of unprotected sex with an infected partner, a teen woman has a 30 percent risk of getting genital herpes. A condom is your best protection against infection. But if you do get herpes, avoid all sexual contact during an outbreak. Don't share towels (or eating utensils if you have mouth sores). And if you've *ever* had a genital herpes infection, use condoms—*even when you can't see sores* (you're infectious a few days before they appear). Also, if you feel discomfort in the area where the sores appear, use a condom, because the pain may mean an outbreak is on the way. Keep using condoms during an attack until sores are crusted over.

TIMING: The infection can remain dormant for months, years, or even life. But if symptoms occur, they generally show within 1 to 3 weeks of infection, lasting an equal amount of time. However, they may then go underground after that first outbreak. About 75 percent of people *will* have reoccurrence, lasting 3 days to 2 weeks each time.

IF UNTREATED: The worst danger is severe discomfort.

TREATMENT: No known cure, but it can be controlled to a certain extent with medication (prescribed by your doctor), which may make the sores come back less often and shorten the time they're around when they do return.

PUBIC LICE ("CRABS")

WHAT: Tiny blood-sucking insects.

HOW: Usually by close contact with an infested person. But you can also get it by sharing towels or bed sheets.

SYMPTOMS: Tiny white balls around your pubic area, underarms, head, eyebrows, and even lashes—any place you have body hair. These eggs hatch into lice, pinhead-sized grayish white clawed creatures (unless they've just finished a meal; then they're dark red). You'll soon experience severe itching, especially at night.

PROTECTION: Dry-clean materials that you think may carry scabies (mini mites that infect your skin) or pubic lice, for example, bedding, towels, and clothing.

TIMING: The lice hatch 7 to 9 days after infection, although you may not notice itching for a few weeks.

IF UNTREATED: Your genitals will continue itching and you may experience rashes.

TREATMENT: A prescribed shampoo for the pubic area. You'll need to sterilize sheets, towels, and toilet seats against reinfection.

SYPHILIS

(SIFF-i-lis)

WHAT: A bacterial infection of the genitals.

HOW: Having unprotected vaginal, oral, or anal sex.

SYMPTOMS: A painless red sore at the place where your body came into contact with the bacteria. Later, headaches, rash, or fever.

PROTECTION: Condoms, though not 100 percent effective.

TIMING: 3 weeks to 8 months after infection.

IF UNTREATED: The syphilis organism—*spirochete*—can remain in the body for life and lead to disfigurement, nerve damage, mental illness, even death.

TREATMENT: Antibiotics.

TRICHOMONIASIS ("TRICH")

(trick-oh-mo-NEYE-ah-sis)

WHAT: An infection of the vagina caused by a parasite.

HOW: Having unprotected vaginal sex.

Are You Infected?

These are the top five signs of an STD:

1 Discharge or bad smell from the vagina or your partner's genitals

2 Pain in the pelvic area

3 Burning or itching around the vagina

4 Vaginal bleeding (other than your period)

5 Major pain during intercourse

If you have any of these symptoms, go to a doctor. Contact Planned Parenthood (see "Address Book" on page 260) for a doctor who will definitely treat you confidentially.

SYMPTOMS: Most people don't have any. Some women may notice a green-yellow frothy vaginal discharge and itching.

PROTECTION: Condoms, though not 100 percent effective.

TIMING: 4 to 20 days after exposure.

IF UNTREATED: "Trich" has no serious long-term consequences, but because it causes major irritation to the vaginal walls, it can increase your chances of catching HIV.

TREATMENT: Antibiotics for both you and your partner.

What does it mean to have safe sex?

DR. MARLIN: Generally, safe sex means your boyfriend wears a condom on his penis during sex so that neither of you get infected with an STD and you don't get pregnant. It's also smart sex. More than half of sexually active teens use condoms. Women can be extra safe by using spermicide in addition to a condom.

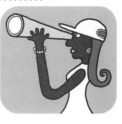

Is AIDS only a gay disease?

DR. MARLIN: Absolutely not. As a female, you are twice as likely to be infected from having sex with a guy who is infected than a guy would be from sleeping with a girl who is infected. The only protection is not having sex or always using a condom correctly, though this is not 100 percent effective (see condom tips on pages 93–94).

I have a weird smell down there. Do I have an STD?

DR. MARLIN: Maybe. You're going to smell different at different times of the month. But if the smell is fishy or very foul, or if there's a discharge, you could have an infection. The only way to be sure is to get checked out by a doctor as soon as possible. Untreated infections can lead to sterility and even death (see Chapter 4).

Can you tell if a guy has an STD by looking?

DR. MARLIN: Not always. Nor can he tell if you have one. Some STDs have visible signs (like sores or pimple-like bumps), but most have no symptoms at all. In fact, STDs are less likely to produce symptoms in guys. So always practice safe sex. About one in four teenagers gets an STD every year.

••

My boyfriend has sores on his lips. Will I get herpes if I kiss him?

••

DR. MARLIN: Yes, but not necessarily how you think. There are two types: herpes simplex virus 1 (HSV-1) and herpes simplex virus 2 (HSV-2 or genital herpes). HSV-1 occurs above the waist, usually as cold sores or lesions in the mouth or on the lips and face. HSV-2 occurs below the waist, usually as genital sores. But both can be transmitted by oral sex. So cold sores can wind up on your genitals. Avoid contact with your guy when he has a visible herpes sore.

Protecting Yourself
Getting in (Birth) Control

The best protection against getting pregnant or getting an STD is always abstinence—that is, *not* having intercourse. That doesn't mean you have to be totally sexless. You can kiss and even caress each other safely and still stop before "going all the way" or "having sex." Now here's how to figure out your second-best choice. And remember that effectiveness depends on correct usage, so listen to your gynecologist and read instructions carefully.

CERVICAL CAP

WHAT: Thimble-shaped rubber cap that you fill with spermicide and fit over your cervix.

HOW: Blocks sperm from uterus (where unfertilized egg may be laying in wait).

PROTECTION: 48 hours, no matter how often you make love.

EFFECTIVENESS AGAINST PREGNANCY: 82–84 percent.

PROTECTION AGAINST STDs: None.

WHERE: You need to be fitted by your doctor, gynecologist, or a trained family planning clinic provider. And the fit needs to be checked annually.

COOL: Can be inserted up to 6 hours before sex. Also, it can stay in place for up to 24 hours. Some protection against pelvic inflammatory disease (PID), a general term referring to infections that invade your reproductive system.

UNCOOL: May dislodge during vigorous intercourse. Women with short fingers may have trouble with insertion. It can't be used during your period. Plus it doesn't protect against STDs such as HIV, herpes, or HPV.

HASSLE FACTOR: Medium. Insertion can be a little awkward, and the cap must be kept in place at least 6 hours after intercourse and washed with soap after it is removed.

OPERATING INSTRUCTIONS: Before inserting, check for holes or tears by holding it up to the light. Fill one-third to one-half of the cap with spermicidal jelly or cream. Insert by squeezing the cap between the thumb and index finger, sliding it into your vagina, and pressing the rim around your cervix (feel around the edge to be sure the cervix is completely covered). To remove, press on the rim until the seal on the cervix is broken, tilt the cap, then hook fingers under the rim and pull sideways out of the vagina. After use, wash with mild soap and water, and dry thoroughly; store in a cool, dry, dark place.

MOST COMMON SCREWUP: Putting it in incorrectly.

RELATIONSHIP STAT: It's better if you're in one.

COST: $13–$25 (plus $8 for spermicide) plus cost of exam.

CONDOM (MALE)

WHAT: Latex, polyurethane, or animal tissue balloon-shaped cover placed over erect penis.

HOW: It bags sperm so that it doesn't enter your body.

PROTECTION: Instant.

EFFECTIVENESS AGAINST PREGNANCY: 88–98 percent.

PROTECTION AGAINST STDs: 97 percent, if it's made of latex or polyurethane (animal tissue condoms don't protect against HIV), against all STDs except genital warts, herpes, and crabs.

WHERE: Pharmacy, drugstore, supermarket, family planning clinics, and some school health offices.

Getting Physical

COOL: Latex condoms are the best protection against all STDs. You don't need to see a doctor to use them, and it can be fun trying different kinds—flavored, ribbed, ridged, knobbed, etc. They also help slow down premature ejaculation.

UNCOOL: Can be used only once. Putting it on and taking it off interrupts the moment. Men complain that their sensations and pleasure are reduced. The condom can break if handled incorrectly (the polyurethane ones are thinner and stronger).

HASSLE FACTOR: Low. Can't be put on until he's semi-hard. Must be removed immediately after ejaculation or it may leak. Need a new one each time—never reuse a condom.

OPERATING INSTRUCTIONS: Keep handling to a minimum to prevent tiny tears. Once the penis is erect, place the rolled-up condom over the head, pinching the little bump at the top that's called the reservoir tip—this'll help collect semen. Then unroll the condom all the way down to the base of the penis (if it doesn't unroll, it's on wrong—start over with a new one). The condom must fit snugly.

As soon as he ejaculates, he should pull out, holding the base of the condom to prevent slippage or spillage. To remove, hold the base of the condom (the rolled-up part) with one hand and use the other hand to take it by the tip. Pulling it off by the tip alone not only makes a mess but you could allow for dripping semen. Throw the condom away.

MOST COMMON SCREWUP: Putting it on too early or too late so that you don't get a proper fit, or tearing it when you put it on/take it off. Not checking the condom's expiration date. Also, using with any oily extra—like vaginal creams, yeast infection creams (even if applied a few days before), Vaseline, baby oil, and massage oils—breaks down the latex, making it as effective as a colander. Same goes for storing condoms in hot, sweaty places like pockets or wallets.

RELATIONSHIP STAT: Doesn't matter.

COST: Around 25-50 cents for one, $2 for three, or $12 for ten.

CONDOM (FEMALE)

WHAT: Shaped like an upside-down sock, it's a larger polyurethane version of the male condom with an inner ring that sits over the cervix and an outer ring that lies flat against the labia (vaginal lips).

HOW: Clings to the vagina and cervix, preventing contact with sperm.

PROTECTION: 24 hours.

EFFECTIVENESS AGAINST PREGNANCY: 88–97 percent.

PROTECTION AGAINST STDs: 97 percent except for genital warts, herpes, and crabs.

WHERE: Pharmacy, drugstore, family planning clinics, and some supermarkets.

COOL: Polyurethane is stronger and thinner than latex and protects the entire genital area, so it offers near-total STD and HIV protection. And it can be put in up to 8 hours before sex. It's also good for those who are sensitive to latex. Plus you don't need to see a doctor to get it.

UNCOOL: Can be used only once. Some people feel less sensation because it covers the whole genital area. It's fairly expensive. Plus it can be creepy-looking and it's been reported to squeak.

HASSLE FACTOR: High. Putting it on is complicated, and you have to remove it right after sex. Also, the outer ring can slip inside you during sex.

OPERATING INSTRUCTIONS: Carefully remove the condom from the package. Hold the condom with the open end down. Use the thumb and middle finger to squeeze the flexible ring at the closed end into a narrow oval. With your other hand, spread the lips of your vagina. Insert the ring and sheath into the vagina. Use your index finger to push the ring as far as possible into the vagina. Insert a finger into the condom until it touches the bottom of the ring. Push the ring up past the pubic bone. Make sure the outer ring and part of the sheath are outside the vagina over the vulva. To remove, spread the lips of the vagina with one hand and reach in with the other to grasp the ring between the thumb and middle or index finger, and carefully draw out. Throw the condom away.

MOST COMMON SCREWUP: Putting it on incorrectly, allowing sperm to leak in.

RELATIONSHIP STAT: Doesn't matter.

Getting
Physical

COST: It costs more than the male condom (about $2.50 per pouch).

DEPO-PROVERA

WHAT: An injection of synthetic progestin in your butt or arm every 3 months.

HOW: The hormone seeps into your bloodstream gradually over the next 3 months, causing ovulation to stop.

PROTECTION: 3 months.

EFFECTIVENESS AGAINST PREGNANCY: 99.8 percent.

PROTECTION AGAINST STDs: None.

WHERE: Doctor, gynecologist, or family planning clinic.

COOL: Doctor injects it and you forget about it for a few months. It protects against pregnancy from day 1 if you get the shot during the first 5 days of your period. It also reduces period cramps.

UNCOOL: There's no protection against STDs, and some side effects may be weight gain, irregular bleeding, headaches, and moodiness. It can take up to 18 months for your body to get back to normal once you stop injections.

HASSLE FACTOR: Medium. You need to get reinjected every 3 months and you may forget to go for your next injection.

OPERATING INSTRUCTIONS: A shot in the arm or butt.

MOST COMMON SCREWUP: Forgetting to get your trimonthly shot.

RELATIONSHIP STAT: Unless you also use a condom, the negative STD protection factor means it's safer if you use this when you're in one relationship.

COST: $30–$75 per shot (you'll need four per year) plus $35–$125 for the initial exam.

DIAPHRAGM

WHAT: A shallow cup you fill with spermicidal cream or jelly and insert up to 6 hours before having sex.

HOW: Prevents sperm from entering uterus.

PROTECTION: 24 hours.

EFFECTIVENESS AGAINST PREGNANCY: 90 percent.

PROTECTION AGAINST STDs: Low.

WHERE: You need to be fitted by your doctor, gynecologist, or a trained family planning clinic provider. And the fit needs to be checked annually.

COOL: Some protection against PID, chlamydia, gonorrhea, and trichomoniasis. It reduces risk of cervical cancer. It can be inserted up to 6 hours before sex.

UNCOOL: It takes practice to put the diaphragm in. You have to be fitted for the right size every year. It has a higher rate of urinary tract infections (UTIs), must be left in place 6 hours after ejaculation, and offers little to no protection against STDs. Also, any oily products (like Vaseline, baby oil, and massage oils) are a no-no as they can make your rubber cup leaky.

HASSLE FACTOR: Medium. You have to add more cream/jelly every time he is going to ejaculate (which in itself can be pretty messy stuff), regularly check for holes, and get it refitted if you gain/lose a lot of weight.

OPERATING INSTRUCTIONS: Before inserting, check for holes or tears by holding it up to the light. Then spread spermicidal jelly or cream on the inside portion of the dome and rim with clean hands. Put the diaphragm all the way back against the cervix, with the cavity containing the spermicide covering the cervical opening; feel around the edge to be sure the cervix is completely covered. If you have sex more than an hour after inserting a diaphragm, or if you have sex more than once, you need to squirt some more spermicide into your vagina (don't remove the diaphragm). Leave the diaphragm in place for at least 6 hours after his last ejaculation, but no more than 24 hours. Remove it by sticking your fingers into your vagina and gently grasping the rim and pulling. Then wash it with soap and water, dry it, and store it in a cool, dry, dark place.

MOST COMMON SCREWUP: Forgetting to add more spermicide.

RELATIONSHIP STAT: The negative STD protection factor means it's safer if you use this when you're in one relationship.

COST: $13–$25 plus cost of exam.

IMPLANTS (NORPLANT)

WHAT: Six match-sized capsules, usually inserted into the arm.

HOW: Causes ovulation to stop for up to 5 years.

Getting Physical

PROTECTION: 5 years.

EFFECTIVENESS AGAINST PREGNANCY: 99.6 percent.

PROTECTION AGAINST STDs: None.

WHERE: Inserted by your doctor, gynecologist, or a trained family planning clinic provider.

COOL: Doctor injects it and you forget about it for the next half decade. It's effective within 24 hours.

UNCOOL: Higher risk of STDs. Removal can be painful and may cause scarring.

HASSLE FACTOR: None.

OPERATING INSTRUCTIONS: The clinician will numb a small area of the arm you use least with a painkiller and then make one small cut to insert the six rod-like capsules. The whole thing takes about 10 minutes and is totally painless. Avoid heavy lifting for a few days. You'll need a follow-up visit within 3 months to make sure that you are not having any problems. Norplant must be removed after 5 years when it stops working (you can get it removed earlier if you want). The procedure to remove the rods is similar to how they are inserted. You can also get restocked when the rods are removed.

MOST COMMON SCREWUP: Forgetting to have it removed or renewed after 5 years.

RELATIONSHIP STAT: Unless you also use a condom, the negative STD protection factor means it's safer if you use this when you're in one relationship.

COST: About $500–$750 for the initial exam and insertion (which works out to be cheaper than birth-control pills over the same time period) and $100–$200 for removal.

COMBINED PILL

WHAT: Two synthetic hormones, estrogen and progestin, in pill form (there are now 45 varieties on the market).

HOW: Prevent ovaries from releasing eggs and alter cervical mucus to block sperm.

PROTECTION: Permanent as long as taking the pill.

EFFECTIVENESS AGAINST PREGNANCY: 97 percent.

PROTECTION AGAINST STDs: None.

WHERE: Through a prescription from a doctor, gynecologist, or family planning clinic.

COOL: Protection all the time. Makes periods more regular, decreases menstrual cramping and PMS, and reduces risk of endometrial and ovarian cancer.

UNCOOL: Can cause breast tenderness, headaches, nausea/depression, doesn't protect against STDs, can't be used if you smoke. You need to know your family history because you may not be able to take it if there's high blood pressure, heart problems, or breast and/or ovarian cancer in your family. Can be unreliable for rest of month if missed even once or if you're sick (if you're puking and/or have the runs, your body's ability to absorb the pill is decreased).

HASSLE FACTOR: Low. You must remember to take it daily around the same time. You'll need backup contraception for the first month as it takes 3–4 weeks before it's effective.

OPERATING INSTRUCTIONS: Swallow.

MOST COMMON SCREWUP: Forgetting to take it (if you do skip a pill, take two the next day *and* use added protection—like a condom—for the rest of the month). Also, forgetting to get refills—don't wait until you run out. Instead, ask your doctor for a refillable prescription and get it rebooted before the end of your current pack.

RELATIONSHIP STAT: Unless you also use a condom, the negative STD protection factor means it's safer if you use this when you're in one relationship.

COST: $15–$25 per month plus $30–$125 for the initial exam.

MINI-PILL

WHAT: The synthetic hormone progestin in pill form.

HOW: Alters cervical mucus to block sperm and prevents fertilized eggs from being implanted in the uterus.

PROTECTION: Permanent as long as taking the pill.

EFFECTIVENESS AGAINST PREGNANCY: 97.5 percent.

PROTECTION AGAINST STDs: None.

WHERE: Through a prescription from a doctor, gynecologist, or family planning clinic.

COOL: Offers protection all the time with less side effects than the combo pill.

UNCOOL: May cause spotting between periods, weight gain, and breast tenderness. No protection against STDs. Can be unreliable for rest of the month if missed even once, and you'll need backup contraception for the first month as it takes 3–4 weeks before it's effective. You need to know your family history because you may not be able to take it if there's high blood pressure, heart problems, or breast and/or ovarian cancer in your family.

HASSLE FACTOR: Low. You must remember to take daily at the same time.

OPERATING INSTRUCTIONS: Swallow.

MOST COMMON SCREWUP: Forgetting to take it at the right time.

RELATIONSHIP STAT: Unless you also use a condom, the negative STD protection factor means it's safer if you use this when you're in one relationship.

COST: $15–$25 per month plus $30–$125 for the initial exam.

SPERMICIDE

WHAT: Creams, foams, jellies, contraceptive films, foaming vaginal tablets, or suppositories that kill sperm before it reaches an egg. Spermicide is most effective when used with diaphragms and cervical caps. It can be used with condoms as well to increase protection.

HOW: Killer chemicals are released when spermicide is inserted 10 minutes to 1 hour before sex.

PROTECTION: Up to 1 hour after application.

EFFECTIVENESS AGAINST PREGNANCY: 79 percent.

PROTECTION AGAINST STDs: None.

WHERE: Pharmacy, drugstore, or supermarket.

COOL: Inexpensive and easy to buy, available without a prescription.

UNCOOL: High STD risk. It can cause irritation in some people.

HASSLE FACTOR: High. Messy, messy, messy; also, except for aerosols, you have to wait 10–15 minutes before having sex and they're only good for an hour, so if you have sex after that, you've got to do the whole thing again.

OPERATING INSTRUCTIONS: For foams, shake container vigorously at least 20–30 times just before insertion. Take careful aim—

you need to have a megadose of spermicide in EXACTLY the right place when he spurts or it doesn't work. For jelly, tablets, suppository, film, or cream, fill the applicator. Lie down and insert the applicator into the vagina until the tip is at or near the cervix; push applicator plunger to release spermicide (after each use, wash applicator with soap and water). Film must be folded in half and inserted with dry fingers near the cervix, or the film will stick to the fingers and not the cervix. Putting about a dab of spermicide gel or cream on his penis right before putting a condom on can boost protection. Use more spermicide each time you have sex.

MOST COMMON SCREWUP: Having sex too soon after application.

RELATIONSHIP STAT: Unless you also use a condom, the negative STD protection factor means it's safer if you use this when you're in one relationship.

COST: $8 per tube.

. . . .

How can I talk to my mother about birth control?

. . . .

DR. MARLIN: Most moms have incredibly mixed feelings about this. It means facing the fact that their daughter is doing grown-up things—like enjoying sex or thinking about enjoying sex. Moms may worry that asking questions means you're going to *do* something.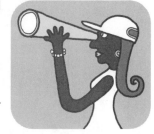

For a daughter, it means thinking about your mother as a sexual being, not just a source of information.

First, choose your time wisely. The night before she has a big presentation to give or the afternoon of your family's 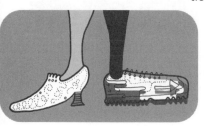 holiday party are *not* good times. Make sure you have privacy and your mom's full attention. Try something like, "Mom, I want to talk to you about something, but I don't want you to panic or worry. Okay?" Wait until she nods her head or answers.

10 Things Your Parents Can't Handle About Your Having Sex

1 That you're having it, part one—it means you really are growing up.

2 That you're having it, part two—as much as they love you, they may be jealous of your opportunities and youth (it reminds them they're getting older).

3 That you're having it, part three—parents have a tough time seeing their kids as sexual beings.

4 That you might make the same mistakes they did.

5 That you might enjoy it.

6 That you won't enjoy it.

7 That you might not be able to handle it emotionally.

8 That you could get pregnant or get an STD.

9 That acknowledging your interest in sex is like giving you a green light to engage in it.

10 That they don't know enough to advise you.

Then say, "I want to have a discussion with you about birth control. This isn't about me having sex. I just want to know the facts and thought you could help me learn how to be responsible and safe about my choices." Hopefully, she will respect your mature attitude and match it.

The Real Sex Facts

What your parents think: The minute you hit your teens, you gotta have it.

The truth: More than half of teenagers are virgins until age 17 and nearly one in five don't have sex at all during adolescence.

What your parents think: Most adults believe the teen pregnancy rate has risen since 1980.

The truth: The number has decreased by 15 percent.

What your parents think: Teens are responsible for most out-of-marriage births.

The truth: They actually account for only 31 percent.

What your parents think: Almost 60 percent of adults believe teens are responsible for most unplanned pregnancies.

The truth: Teens account for 23 percent of those pregnancies.

What your parents think: Adults guess that 53 percent of teens use contraception.

The truth: About 93 percent of sexually active girls report using some sort of birth control, usually the male condom (though not always correctly or consistently).

LAURA: I'm lucky because I don't have to worry about having a talk with her. We're writing this book together! We've been talking about sex for years, so it's never one big deal here-we-go kind of thing.

I heard about a girl who wanted to talk to her mother about birth control but thought her mother would freak out. So she talked to her mother's cool aunt, who talked to her mom, and that eased her into it. A lot of my friends talk to my mother. So find someone older and knowledgeable to talk to you if you can't talk to your mom. You don't want this to be an unpleasant discussion. Sex should be pleasurable and you shouldn't feel ashamed.

....

I'm pregnant. I don't even know how to tell my boyfriend, let alone my parents.

....

DR. MARLIN: You're going to need your parents in many ways: emotionally, financially, logistically, medically, legally (see "Getting an Abortion" on page 109).

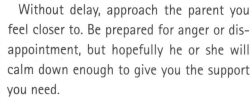

Without delay, approach the parent you feel closer to. Be prepared for anger or disappointment, but hopefully he or she will calm down enough to give you the support you need.

Telling the guy is the test of boyfriendhood: If he can't face it, he really can't come through at one of the most important times in your life. And what does that tell you?

LAURA: As close as I am to my mom, I'd have a tough time doing this. She would feel like a failure after all the information and help she's given me.

But I also think your friends are not the ones who necessarily have the best advice on how to deal with it. They're full of sympathy, but they believe crazy stuff, like if you drink cola in the bath you'll lose the baby.

So find someone outside the situation to confide in and give you advice and a neutral point of view. A lot of kids in my school trust the school nurse. She won't let them miss classes without a good reason, but she's also very sympathetic. Another friend goes to her church's peer group where there's an advisor who helps deal with tough issues.

....

My boyfriend swears he can control himself so that we don't need condoms.

....

DR. MARLIN: This is one of those know-your-limits times. First, arm yourself with facts. The time it takes a male to go from erection to ejaculation is about 2 minutes. And it takes even less time for a young person. So it's unlikely that your boyfriend will be able to control himself as he says.

Also, when a guy is sexually excited, he leaks a clear fluid *before* he ejaculates. Even a micro-drop contains sperm that can swim in the moisture outside the vagina to the fallopian tubes, where fertilization occurs.

Find ways to make using condoms sexy.

Try stroking his penis from the tip to the base as you roll the condom on.

No matter how much he controls himself, *you can still get pregnant or get an STD.* So use birth control. It's called protection for a reason.

LAURA: You may not be able to convince him. But it's a simple problem and doesn't take a long discussion—no love without the glove.

LAURA'S TIP: Here's why I will not have sex without using birth control: A friend thought she was pregnant. She worried about (1) raising a child at age 16, (2) disappointing and shaming her family, and (3) being kicked out of school (her school kicked out women who became pregnant, but the fathers were allowed to stay). She also had to decide if she should tell her family and her boyfriend before she knew for sure. And if she was pregnant, should she have an abortion, keep the baby, or put it up for adoption?

We had long talks. Friends said they would help if she decided to keep the baby, but this was unrealistic. What could we do besides be there for her? Giving her our spending money wouldn't go far, and I know from babysitting that most of us were just thinking about the fun part of looking after a baby—not when it cries or gets sick, not to mention that babies need round-the-clock care. Then there's the loss of sleep, neglect of studies, and cost of raising a child (as my mother constantly reminds me, the average is $150,000 for the first 18 years).

Luckily she wasn't pregnant, but all this worry could have been avoided if she had used birth control.

··

I want to get on the pill, but I don't know how. I can't ask my parents.

··

DR. MARLIN: If you don't feel comfortable going to your family doctor (although they are legally supposed to treat your request confidentially, some doctors don't adhere to this), Planned Parenthood will provide affordable, confidential reproductive health care and sexual health information (see "Address Book" on page 260).

LAURA: The kids in my school don't use the pill because it doesn't protect against STDs, and girls worry about what it will do to their bodies. They use condoms because they're safe, you can get them from the drugstore, and the school nurse gives them out.

··

There are so many different kinds of condoms. How can I choose a good one?

··

DR. MARLIN: Always go for a brand name with FDA (Food and Drug Administration) approval. One study put more than 30 brands to a stretch test and found that Ramses Sensitol, Gold Circle Coin, Gold Circle, Sheik Classic, and Durex Nuform had the least leakage and breakage.

Using a condom is easy, but the first time can be tricky. Try it at home first without the pressure of your boyfriend watching (you can practice on a banana), and get your boyfriend to practice on himself. Either or both of you can put the condom on him at the right time, so both of you should know how (see pages 93–94 for more on how to use a condom correctly).

....

Help—the condom broke!

....

DR. MARLIN: Luckily, a few options can reduce your chance of pregnancy by as much as 90 percent. These treatments block pregnancy. They are *not* the same thing as an abortion, which terminates pregnancy.

Get your doctor to prescribe emergency contraceptive pills (ECPs). You can also get them from Planned Parenthood or they can direct you to a doctor who can prescribe them. These high-dose birth-control pills must be taken within 72 hours of unprotected sex (followed by a second dose 12 hours later), so you can't waste any time.

There are some side effects—temporary breast tenderness, nausea and vomiting—but those are mild compared to pregnancy.

You can take a specific dose of mini-pills (birth-control pills that contain only the progestin hormone). These should be taken within 48 hours after unprotected sex (again, followed by a second dose 12 hours later).

Have your doctor insert an intrauterine device (IUD). You can do this up to 7 days after unprotected sex. Insertion may hurt a bit, but it will protect from pregnancy. It can be removed after your doctor has given you clearance (generally after your period).

None of these treatments can prevent disease. So wash your vagina—inside and out—with mild soap and water. But don't douche because it can increase your chances of getting a pelvic inflammatory disease. Also, getting tested for STDs is a good idea. Next time, for the absolute best protection against both pregnancy and STDs, use (1) a latex condom *plus* (2) a separate spermicide *plus* (3) backup contraception such as the pill or a diaphragm.

....

The condom is missing. I think it's stuck in me.

....

DR. MARLIN: Wash your hands and stick your pointer and middle fingers into your vagina to see if you can feel it (think of it as inserting a tampon, only going in deeper). If you can, carefully pull the condom out and throw it away. Then go ASAP to the doctor (call Planned Parenthood for information on where to get emergency contraception [EC] to prevent pregnancy; see previous question for information on how EC works).

DR. MARLIN'S TIP: Action-packed sex can sometimes make a condom slide up to the top of the penis and slip off. But more often, it's because it was put on incorrectly. Make sure he's erect before you put the condom on. And take it off by holding the rim of the condom as soon as he ejaculates (see condom tips on pages 93–94).

How can I tell if I'm pregnant?

DR. MARLIN: If you had unprotected sex, that's a clue. You might miss your period or your blood flow might be lighter than usual, your breasts might be tender, you might need to urinate more often, or you might feel nauseous, extra hungry, or tired. However, you may not have these symptoms.

The only way to be sure is to take a pregnancy test. There are easy-to-use kits (you urinate onto a stick and the results show up) at the drugstore for around $8 that you can use 2 weeks after unprotected sex, the day after you miss your period, or if your period is on time but different in some way—heavier, lighter, earlier, later. The test can give a false negative result—meaning you may be pregnant, but the test indicates you are not—if you use marijuana.

He came all over me. Can I get pregnant?

DR. MARLIN: Definitely. Even if he ejaculated just on the outside of your vagina—if he was rubbing against it, for instance—sperm can still make its way in. Or if you get sperm on your hands and then touch your vagina, you're also at risk. The only way to safeguard against pregnancy is to make sure your naked genitals don't come in contact with his sperm at all. So if you're fooling around naked, use a condom, even if you're not planning to have intercourse.

....

Can I get pregnant if I have sex during my period?

....

DR. MARLIN: Your highest risk is when you're ovulating (your ovary releases an egg, usually halfway between the first day of your last period and the first day of your next period), but women get pregnant at all times in their cycle, and it's best to assume no time is safe. Sperm can live in your body 8 days after ejaculation. So if you have unprotected sex at the end of your period and happen to ovulate early, you most certainly can get pregnant. And having your period is never a protection from STDs. So always use protection.

....

I heard that you can prevent pregnancy if you wash right after he climaxes in you.

....

DR. MARLIN: You heard wrong. It doesn't do a thing to kill sperm. And it's also possible to get pregnant if it is your first time having sex, if he pulls out too abruptly, if you're really young, or if you have sex right before, during, or after your period.

The only thing that prevents pregnancy is using effective birth control every time you have sex.

DR. MARLIN'S TIP: Washing afterward is a good idea for cutting down on urinary tract infections and STDs that condoms don't protect you from (such as genital warts, herpes, and crabs).

Getting an Abortion

Abortion is a way to end pregnancy. According to the most recent statistics, 20 of every 1,000 women ages 15–44 will have an abortion this year.

You have the right to an abortion, but depending on the state in which you live, you may have to jump through some legal hoops to get one. If you are under 18, you may have to notify one or both of your parents and/or get their consent (even if they're divorced), have a "cooling off" period before you make your decision, or be denied an abortion if you are more than 6 weeks into your pregnancy.

Many doctors no longer perform abortions, either because of their own beliefs or because they have been harassed by anti-abortion groups. See "Abortion: Where to Go" on page 111 for information on finding a sympathetic, competent doctor.

How is an abortion performed?

DR. MARLIN: The safest, easiest, and fastest procedure is dilation and curettage (D&C). It takes a few hours and doesn't require a stay in the hospital (some doctors do it right in their office). You will be given an anesthetic and won't feel a thing during the operation (although afterward you may have cramping, some pelvic pain, and period-like bleeding). The cervix is expanded (dilated) and the endometrial lining of the uterus (the stuff you shed every month with your period) is removed along with the embryo.

It can take your cervix up to 3 weeks to close again, so to reduce the risk of infection you won't be able to take baths, swim, use tampons, and have intercourse during that time. You'll bleed for around 2 to 3 weeks and might feel some cramping. See "Abortion: What to Expect" on page 112.

I'm pregnant and I think I want to keep the baby.

DR. MARLIN: Consider the time and commitment involved in raising a child as a single parent in her teens. Are you ready to take this leap into adult responsibility? Will keeping the baby interfere with your goals? Did you plan to finish high school? How about going to college? Will you have financial and emotional support if you keep the baby?

Have you thought about getting up in the middle of the night to take care of the baby? Or not getting any sleep at all? Or living with someone who cries all the time and can't tell you what's wrong? Having to stay home while your friends are out having fun?

Getting
Physical

Younger mothers are more likely to drop out of high school and have a higher rate of divorce, lower paying jobs, and express less satisfaction with their lives.

If you decide to have an abortion, the earlier the better. Fewer than 1 percent of women who undergo legal abortion experience serious complication. But the longer you wait, the more complicated and traumatic (and expensive) the experience is going to be.

Rape

In the next 2 minutes, a woman in the United States will be raped. If she's like 75 percent of rape victims, she will know her attacker.

Abortion: What to Expect

There are three types of abortions. The procedure depends on when during the pregnancy you have it done:

1. Medical abortions use a combination of drugs up to 49 days after the first day of the last menstrual period to end the pregnancy. There's no surgery. First you get an injection or you're given pills to swallow. A few days later, you insert the medication in tablet form into your vagina. The pregnancy usually ends at home anywhere within 4 hours to a day or two. The embryo and other products of conception that develop during pregnancy are passed through the vagina. The contents look like a heavy period.

   Advantages: Anesthesia is not required, no surgical instruments are used, the experience resembles a very bad period, the procedure is relatively private, and it can be provided very early in pregnancy.

   Disadvantages: Not as widely available as surgical abortion, it may take as long as a few weeks to complete, and it requires three visits to the doctor. Bleeding lasts a few weeks. You may see the fetus when it aborts from your body. Side effects can include nausea, headache, weakness, cramping, and fatigue. One to 12 percent of medical abortions fail, and then surgical procedures are required to end the pregnancy.

2. Surgical abortions are the most common kind. They can be done with the gentle suction of a syringe, which is called manual vacuum aspiration (MVA), or with a suction device, from the time you suspect you're pregnant up to about 14 weeks from your last period.

The procedure takes about 10 to 20 minutes. The vagina is washed with an antiseptic. Usually, a local anesthetic is injected into or near the cervix. The opening of the cervix is gradually stretched. One after the other, a series of increasingly thick rods (dilators) are inserted into the opening. The dilators absorb fluids and stretch the opening of the cervix.

After the cervix opening is stretched, a tube attached to a suction machine is inserted through it into the uterus to gently suck out the contents of the uterus. To be sure that the uterus has been completely emptied after the suction tube has been removed, a curette (narrow metal loop) may be used to gently scrape the walls of the uterus.

Advantages: The procedure is quick, generally only two visits to the doctor are required (including one for follow-up), and side effects are similar to a normal period.

Disadvantages: The procedure requires the use of invasive instruments, cannot normally be performed in very early stages of pregnancy, is less effective after 7 weeks of pregnancy, and bleeding lasts a few days to a week.

3. Abortions after 14 weeks of pregnancy are available in some clinics and hospitals up to the 24th week of pregnancy. After that, it's almost impossible to get an abortion—the procedure has become a political flash point, and even if your state allows it (right now, 17 don't, except when your life is truly in danger), many doctors won't do it.

Rape, legally defined as a sexual act committed against a woman's will, has far more to do with power and emotional imbalance than it does with sex.

....

I was attacked and raped last year on my way home from work. No one knows. I thought I had recovered, but I've been reliving what happened and I'm even scared to kiss my boyfriend.

....

DR. MARLIN: Rape is a terrible violation of your body and of your trust in everyone. I know. I was raped, too. In college, by a boy I knew. I never reported it. I thought somehow I had brought it on myself—they didn't have the term *date rape* back then.

Keeping my pain inside only made it worse. It took years to recover from feeling ashamed, from the loss of trust in other people, and from my lack of confidence in my ability to take care of myself. I had problems with sex for a long time and felt angry, sad, and alone.

Make sure your partner knows about your experience and understands you may need to pull back during sexual activity if you get upset. Healing is a long process. Give yourself room and be sure the partners you choose can allow you that room. It also helped me to talk to a trained counselor.

Rape can make you feel helpless, but you can take control of the situation. If you don't want to get involved in a court case, you can still file a report. This

You've Been Raped If...

❋ Your body has been touched or penetrated in any way against your will.
❋ You have made it clear you don't want to be touched.
❋ You said yes, then changed your mind and said no in the middle of getting sexually involved with someone and that person didn't stop.
❋ You are forced to have sex against your will.
❋ You are persuaded to have sex against your will.
❋ You are threatened to have sex against your will.

Protect Yourself

Rapists prey on people they perceive as weak. So the more active you are about your safety, the less likely you'll be seen as a target:

❁ Take elevators (stairwells are more dangerous). And get off if you feel uncomfortable when someone gets on.

❁ Stand with your back to the wall while waiting for a train, meeting a friend outside, or wherever you are. Otherwise, a rapist could sneak up behind you and grab you when your guard is down.

❁ Don't answer the door for a strange woman or man. The woman could be a front for a dangerous man.

❁ If you feel you are in danger, call the police. Dial 911 or 0 for the operator.

❁ Don't stay alone with a man in a room, apartment, or car if you feel uncomfortable—even if you know him.

❁ Limit your drinking and don't take drugs. Alcohol can play a big role in date rape: One study found 55 percent of female students and 75 percent of male students involved in such a rape had been drinking or using drugs (alcohol decreases motor skills, making it difficult to protect yourself, while making a man more sexually aggressive and more likely to take a "no" for a "yes" or a "maybe").

❁ Follow your intuition. If a situation feels bad, get out of it. Don't worry about looking silly or hurting a guy's feelings.

❁ Always keep an eye on your drink, don't take drinks from strangers, and never leave your drink unattended.

❁ Tell people where you're going. It is always wise to let someone know where you'll be and when you plan to come home. You can even log onto www.smartdate.com and register your whereabouts, so if something goes wrong you can be traced.

10-Step Plan to Stop a Rapist in His Tracks

If a guy you're with tries to force you to have sex, here are some things you can try to stop him:

1 Stay calm and think. How serious is he? What options do you have? Is it safe to resist? Women who quickly fight, scream, claw, and gouge have a much better chance of stopping the rape than those who beg, plead, and cry—because rape has as much to do with dominance and power as sex.

2 Say "No!" strongly and with certainty. Don't leave any doubt. Don't worry about being polite.

3 Use the word "rape." This sometimes shocks an attacker into realizing what he's doing and stopping it: "This is rape—stop it!"

4 Assess the situation. Can you escape? Are there people around to help?

is not the same as pressing charges. Filing a report means going to the police to state what happened for the record; pressing charges means actually taking your case to court. If you do press charges, you can change your mind and withdraw your case at any time. *You* are in control of the police process.

If you file a report, the police will ask questions and urge you to visit a hospital for an evidence collection exam. A detective will ask you to describe the assault in detail. Many victims find this invasive, but it's necessary for finding and arresting the right person. The detective will approach your attacker and decide whether to make an arrest and (if you so desire) press charges.

5 Find an escape route. If you can distract him, you might be able to get away.

6 Act quickly. The longer you stay, the fewer your options.

7 Fight back physically. Punch, kick, hit him with any available object and run away fast.

8 You can also shout "Fire!" But do not shout "Help!" Many people will not want to get involved, but fire threatens everyone and you're more likely to get assistance.

9 Tell him you have AIDS, herpes, or some other STD, you're pregnant, or that someone you know will be coming soon.

10 If he's armed, attempt to talk him out of it. If possible, distract him so you can run away, but only if you're sure you have a reasonable chance of escape.

Getting Physical

LAURA: It makes me angry that women have to worry about rape while men don't—every time my girlfriends and I go out on our own, this is something we think about. If there is a stranger on the street looking at me in a weird way, I need to decide whether moving away makes me more or less of a target because I look strong or afraid. If I hear a noise behind me while walking alone, should I be concerned?

None of my guy friends worry about these things.

LAURA'S TIP: It might help you to listen to Tori Amos. She was raped and she wrote songs to help her deal with it. Her CD *Little Earthquakes* has at least two songs, "Little Earthquakes" and "Silent All These Years,"

If You've Been Raped

* Immediately go to a friend or family member you trust who can be with you indefinitely (if you think you've been drugged, you have 4 to 12 hours to be tested for the presence of drugs).
* As much as you want to take a shower, don't until after you contact the police, make a report, and are tested. Showering can remove evidence like semen, skin and hair, clothing fibers, and fingerprints.
* Start recalling details about your attacker (hair color, height and weight, clothing, skin color, scars and tattoos, etc.), any vehicle (license plate, make, model, color, dents), and location, and write these down.
* Call the police or go with someone you trust to the station to report a rape. You should state as soon as pos-

that many rape victims have found comforting. She also helped set up the Rape, Abuse & Incest National Network (RAINN) for rape victims (see "Address Book" page 259).

The Healing Process

It can take years to recover from being raped. The most important thing is not to blame yourself. You may have walked home alone against your better judgment, you may have been at a party and had too much to drink, or you may have gone off alone with someone who you trusted, then changed your mind, or been sexually engaged with someone and then decided you did not want to continue. *Even so, if you have not given consent, the rape was not your fault.*

Here are some of the emotions you may go through if you have been raped:

sible that you wish to prosecute. You can change your mind later, but saying so will initiate testing and careful reporting of the incident. Do not at any point appear to waver on your desire to prosecute, even if you are unsure. If you do decide to go ahead with prosecution, your uncertainty could eventually be used against you by the defendant during the trial.

* Ask for a rape crisis counselor or advocate for help and support during this process.
* Seek medical attention as soon as possible after you have been tested (rape testing is usually done at the hospital, and you can get tested for STDs and receive emergency contraception for pregnancy at the same time).
* Talk to someone trained in rape counseling to begin your healing.

Fear: Here's how it may play out:

* You become fearful of unfamiliar situations and distrust new acquaintances and even old friends.
* You may have trouble getting into new relationships, especially if your rapist was someone you trusted.
* You have difficulty communicating your needs to your partners.
* You fear sex.

Guilt: Victims often feel they somehow may have provoked the rape or that they should have done something to stop it.

Anger: Anger is healthy. You have been treated as an object. You may feel rage over being deceived and betrayed if you knew the assailant.

Shame/embarrassment: Our bodies are private. You may feel embarrassment at having to repeat the details to police and other strangers.

Loss of control: Rape victims are forced to submit against their will. You need reassurance that you're capable of making effective decisions and assuming control over your life again. About one-third of victims suffer from depression, thoughts of suicide, and/or drug/alcohol abuse.

All these reactions are normal. Healing often requires help from many people, including friends, family, counselors, and support groups, to learn to cope with feelings of anger, shame, loss of trust, powerlessness, depression, and self-blame.

Date-Rape Drugs

There have been increasing incidents of guys slipping tasteless drugs like gamma hydroxy butyrate, or GHB (a homemade illegal tranquilizer) in women's drinks. The drugs induce deep sleep and cause memory loss, making anyone who unwittingly ingests them an easy target. The effects begin in 30 minutes, peak within 2 hours, and may persist for up to 8 hours or more, depending upon dosage.

If you suspect a date-rape drug was used in an assault, it is important to get tested within 4 to 8 hours, 12 hours for urine tests. Date-rape drugs leave the system very rapidly.

One Last Sex Tip from Dr. Marlin

The decision to have sex or not, and when, is a personal one that only you can make. Your boyfriend shouldn't make the decision for you and it is not something to be used as a weapon to hurt your parents. Your first time is something you always remember. If the experience is good, you will tend to have good relationships and good sexual experiences the rest of your life. And if the experience is bad, it may color everything afterward.

Bear in mind that 30 percent of people never have sex again with the partner they lose their virginity to. Only about 25 percent of

Alert

Keep your eye out for these things while dating:

* He doesn't listen to you, ignores you, or talks over you: This shows that he has little respect for you and might not buy it when you say "no."
* He gets into your personal space, making you feel uncomfortable: You don't need to have some creep pawing you.
* He says negative things about women: It's a small jump from hostile feelings to violent acts, particularly when alcohol is involved.
* He does what he wants regardless of your wishes: If he makes all the decisions about where to go and what to do without asking your opinion, he may not care whether you want to have sex.
* He plays on your guilt when you don't give him what he wants: If he calls you uptight or a prude, don't let it get to you. Remember, he just wants sex and doesn't care about your feelings.
* He acts possessive or jealous if you mention a male friend: Bad news. Guys like this usually have a bad temper.
* He drinks heavily: If he's rejected, he may get angry and violent and try to force sex on you.

women report enjoying first intercourse physically, and less than 8 percent report orgasm from first intercourse. Those numbers most likely result from being ill-prepared, simply not knowing the basics, and having unrealistic expectations.

Imagine you're standing on the edge of a diving board, 100 feet above the pool. If you're ready to try diving, you've learned what to do, and you really want to do it, your mind and body will cooperate.

You probably won't execute the perfect dive the first time, but you'll feel good, and you won't hurt yourself. On the other hand, if you're not ready, you don't know how, or you don't want to, your body and mind just won't let you. Your feet will keep inching back, your heart will race, your head will say "No, no, no," and you just won't be able to.

That's a good thing: Our bodies and minds work together to keep us safe.

4
Getting Powerful

Adolescence is the time when your body becomes sexually mature. You start producing and releasing hormones that trigger physical changes. Exactly when these changes begin depends on your own body's schedule. Puberty in girls usually starts between ages 8 and 13. In guys, it normally occurs between ages 10 and 15.

During puberty, you gain weight and grow hair under your arms and around your vagina. Your body gets curvier as you develop breasts and hips and have your first period.

Guys get more muscular, their voices become deeper, their penises widen and lengthen, and they also develop hair under their arms and around their penises.

One of the hardest things about puberty is timing. Not knowing when and how your body will change causes anxiety. You worry if you haven't started your period as soon as your friends, or that you will be terminally flat-chested. Or you may be uncomfortable if you're the first to use tampons and wear a bra. Eventually, however, everyone catches up, and the differences between you and your friends even out.

Puberty

All my friends have periods and are getting breasts. I feel like their little sister. Help!

DR. MARLIN: Don't worry—it will happen. The pace of puberty tends to be genetic. If you're late, your mother and sisters probably were too, which may make them a good source for advice on how to deal with the frustration.

You will not be stuck in pre-puberty long. So mellow out. You're going through something remarkable, and each stage is to be savored, not dreaded or rushed.

LAURA: When my friends and I started growing breasts and getting taller, we'd measure ourselves obsessively. At first, I was really jealous. I almost cried the day my best friend got her period and I didn't have mine yet. But it turned out to be a good thing because I got a chance to see how she dealt with the changes and knew what to expect without having to figure it out while I was experiencing it.

Do guys freak about their bodies the way girls do?

DR. MARLIN: Absolutely. Their voices are breaking, they sweat more, they're often shorter than girls the same age, their skin is breaking out worse than yours, and they can't control their erections. They're stressed

His Puberty

The changes a boy's body is going through right now can be separated into five stages, but timing can vary:

Stage 1: *Usually between ages 9 and 12.* Male hormones become active, but there are hardly any outward signs. Testicles are maturing, and some boys start a period of rapid growth late in this stage.

Stage 2: *Usually between ages 9 and 15.* The testicles and scrotum enlarge, but penis size doesn't increase much, and there is very little, if any, pubic hair. Height increases and body shape starts to change.

Stage 3: *Usually between ages 11 and 16.* The penis starts to grow in length but not much in width. The testicles and scrotum are still growing. Pubic hair, darker and coarser, spreads toward the legs. Height growth continues and body/face shape are more adult. The voice begins to deepen (and crack).

Stage 4: *Usually between ages 11 and 17.* Penis width increases, as well as length. The testicles and scrotum keep growing. Pubic hair begins to have adult (wiry, darker) texture. Most boys have their first ejaculations, usually in the form of wet dreams (during sleep) or masturbation. Underarm hair develops. Facial hair increases on the chin and upper lip. The voice gets deeper and the skin more oily.

Stage 5: *Usually between ages 14 and 18.* Males attain full adult height and physique. Pubic hair and genitals have adult appearance. Facial hair grows more.

Getting Powerful

about their penis size in the same way you stew about breasts. They worry about not having enough chest hair or muscles to attract girls.

LAURA'S TIP: It can be cool to talk to your guy friends (not a boyfriend) about what they worry about bodywise. The specifics are different, but they all have items on their freak-out list!

> I have huge breasts. I wear a heavy-duty bra and the straps dig into my shoulders. I'm sick and tired of guys at school trying to feel me up.

DR. MARLIN: If boys touch you without your permission, that's sexual assault. You can report them to the school principal, but that might make the hassling worse. I'd use scare tactics on them and shout in a loud, firm (not hysterical) voice, "Get your hands off me!" Chances are they'll be so startled, they'll back off right away.

Studies show adolescence is harder for girls who develop earlier because they are treated as sexually promiscuous regardless of their behavior. Guys love to look at breasts and it's worse right now when they have all those sex hormones surging throughout their body.

You are going to have to learn how to deal with unwanted attention faster than the other girls in your class. The only way to do that is to believe in yourself. Your breasts, while undoubtedly a hassle, are also a beautiful part of your womanhood. And let's face it, having something everyone else values can be a huge ego booster.

So while you may uncomfortable wearing clothes that accentuate your size, don't hide your breasts either. Make sure you have a properly fitted bra to give you support.

LAURA: You have what every girl wants. Okay, I know that doesn't help you any more than it helps me when people tell me that my dark thick hair is what every girl wants (dark thick hair also means dark hairy legs and underarms).

But isn't it weird that some women spend thousands of dollars to make their breasts bigger and others hate their big breasts and wish they were smaller?

I read somewhere that the perfect breast can fit in a champagne glass. My friends and I tried that—we range from an A to C cup and not one of us could squeeze our boobs in there. It just shows you how screwed up the whole breast size business is.

··

I'm an A cup and my breasts don't seem to have grown since seventh grade. Is this possible? Can I make them bigger?

··

DR. MARLIN: Breasts usually start budding a few years before a girl gets her first period and stop a few years after. Some girls are fully developed by age 14; others don't fully mature until 18 or even 20. So your cleavage may well be coming—the only question is when. On the other hand, some women remain an A cup—but it's probably too early to tell since you haven't finished your growth spurt(s) yet.

Excessive dieting and exercising (2 hours or more of aerobics a day) can cause you to skip periods or stop menstruating altogether. That's a warning sign that your body isn't secreting estrogen, the female hormone, and your breasts can stop growing too.

There is no secret cream to make your breasts bigger. However, you can do bench presses which, although they don't make breasts bigger, develop the muscle under them, making them appear bigger. Wearing a Wonderbra has a similar effect and is much easier.

LAURA: I was surprised to find the average model's size is a B cup. Ads make you think the whole world is a C+ but you.

My breasts are not all that big, but I (sometimes) see it as an advantage. Small breasts screen out stupid guys. I'd rather a guy pick me for me than whether I could work at Hooters. Tell guys like that to go buy a plastic blow-up doll instead. And get yourself a real man—one who is looking for a real woman, not a fantasy plaything.

....
I stink down there. Help!
....

DR. MARLIN: First of all, stop the "down there" stuff. Call things by their proper names. Your body parts are nothing to be ashamed about. Knowing and using the correct words—vagina, in this instance—gives you power and pride in yourself as a woman.

The whole feminine product market helps propagate shame. Your body's smells are a symptom of puberty, your body developing its own unique fragrance. This is what helps attract the opposite sex.

The vagina is self-cleansing and rarely needs to be perfumed or cleaned. In fact, feminine hygiene sprays and douches are at best unnecessary and at worst, can create more smells because they irritate delicate tissues of the vulva and vagina, possibly increasing the chance of vaginal infection. Several studies have linked douching to increased risk of pelvic inflammatory disease, a serious, often fertility-impairing infection of the fallopian tubes.

Soap and water is the best deterrent to vaginal odors. What you wear also has an effect: Nylon underwear, pantyhose, and tight jeans can increase bacteria growth and smells. Cotton and loose outerwear are best.

You may notice liquid coming from your vagina. This is a vaginal secretion, which helps keep it clean. Vaginal secretions generally have an earthy scent. After menstruation, the discharge is thick, white, and waxy; at ovulation it becomes clear and stringy like raw egg white (if it smells fishy or funky, looks cottage cheesy, or is accompanied by itching or burning, you may have an infection).

LAURA: I'm not always crazy about the way I smell, but I can't imagine douching. There's nothing dirty about my sex organs. And I don't want to smell like strawberries or mountain mist. Besides, guys have a scent and I don't hear anyone complaining. Why don't they have penis wipes?

Going to the Gyno

Going to the gynecologist is scary only because you don't know what's going to happen. Here are some tips:

1. Be sure to relax, and use the bathroom first to empty your bladder or bowels so that you don't have to go during the exam (ask if you have to give a urine sample first—you can do that at the same time).
2. The doctor will begin with questions about your medical history that you (and your mother, if she's with you) will answer.
3. You'll then be asked to remove all your clothes and change into a gown.
4. Your doctor may give you a basic physical, including an examination of your eyes and ears, heart and lungs, blood pressure, and weight and a basic abdominal exam, massaging your stomach and hip area, and asking if any spots are tender or painful. The doctor may also take a blood sample from your arm to check hormone levels (which in the case of abnormal periods may be out of whack). You may also get a standard blood and urine screen for STDs.
5. The doctor will do a breast exam, feeling your breasts and chest area to check for lumps, cysts, or other abnormalities. The doctor will also check for discharge from your nipples or anything unusual about the size and shape of your breasts.
6. The pelvic exam is next. It doesn't hurt, although you might feel slightly uncomfortable at some points. It takes about 5 minutes.

    You'll lie on the examining table and put your heels in the little foot holders called stirrups. Your doctor will start by checking your external genitals (or vulva) for cysts and redness, irritation, and discharge. Then she or he will examine your cervix, the opening in your uterus, with a speculum, a sanitary plastic or metal clamp shaped like a duck's bill that is used to hold the vagina open. If you have not had intercourse or stretched the vaginal walls by exploring your body yourself, this may hurt a little bit, but the doctor will use a size that is not too uncomfortable (if

Getting Powerful

you're curious, you can ask for a mirror to see what your cervix looks like when the speculum is in).

A doctor cannot tell who has and who has not had intercourse by the width or tightness of the vagina, or by the state of the hymen. Also, a gynecologist cannot "devirginize" you by examining you.

You may feel some pressure in your bladder (it may feel like you have to suddenly urinate, even if you don't) when the speculum is in, and if you do, let the doctor know to make adjustments so that you are more comfortable.

The doctor will then give you a Pap smear by using a long Q-tip-shaped stick to gently scrape the cervix for cell samples. These will then be tested for the presence of cancerous cells. If you're sexually active, your doctor may also gently scrape off cervical mucus to test for STDs. This scraping doesn't hurt.

For the last part of the exam, your gynecologist will insert one or two gloved, lubricated fingers in your vagina and press gently on your lower abdomen with the other hand to feel internal organs, including your uterus, ovaries, and fallopian tubes. Tell your doctor if you feel any sensitivity or pain because it could indicate an infection, enlarged ovaries or uterus, cysts, or tumors.

Some doctors also examine the area between the rectum and vagina by placing one gloved finger inside your rectum and the other inside your vagina. You may feel pressure—like you're going to have a bowel movement. Don't worry, it's normal and should go away in a few seconds.

That's it. If you have questions, don't hesitate to ask the doctor. If you have any pain during the exam, speak up.

Test results should be back from the lab in a week to 10 days. You're done until next year.

I'm scared to go to the gynecologist. Do I have to?

DR. MARLIN: It's a good idea if any of the following apply to you: if you're having sex, you've gotten your period, you haven't gotten your period by the time you are 16, or no matter what at 18. Think of it as taking good care of yourself.

LAURA: I was really scared the first time. I thought that there would be a dark room with a dirty man with cold metal forceps. But it wasn't bad. Just remember to breathe.

My mom made the appointment for me. I insisted on a woman doctor. And I made my mother come in and hold my hand throughout the entire examination.

First the doctor explained what she was going to do. It all felt very weird to have someone looking at my vagina. I was so focused on what the doctor was doing that I can't even remember what she told me or how I answered her questions. Aside from feeling weird, it didn't hurt at all.

Afterward, I felt I had really crossed a threshold. There's no way I could view myself as a little girl anymore.

LAURA'S TIP: I prefer a woman gynecologist, but I have a friend who says a man is better. She's on the swim team and had a yeast infection, so her mom made an emergency appointment and the only doctor they could find was a guy. Well, she was thrilled: He was young and cute, and my friend couldn't wait to get undressed and show him her stuff (as if he were interested! The examination should be strictly clinical—if it isn't, let someone know immediately).

Another friend says when she was suffering from her period cramps that the first doctor she saw was dismissive, told her to use Motrin, and acted like it was no big deal. But the doctor she now goes to is sympathetic and has given her good dietary advice. So gynecologist gender depends on you. Try different ones and decide how comfortable you feel

Getting Powerful

opening your legs—and thoughts—to a particular doctor. The most important thing is having a good doctor you can trust.

Periods

I haven't gotten my period yet and I'm freaked I'm going to get it at school, or worse, when I'm on a date.

DR. MARLIN: First periods are usually light, just a little brownish spotting. If you forget your just-in-case pad, there are a lot of substitutes: Roll up some toilet paper and wad it in your underwear. Even a sock will do in a pinch. If you stain your underwear, wash the blood out with cold water.

LAURA: I got my period for the first time traveling in California with my father when I was 12. My stomach really hurt (I realized later that these were cramps). We both thought I was having some gastric attack and he took me to the hospital. In the ER I went to the bathroom, saw the blood, and realized what was happening. I tried to think of a way to tell my dad, but I was too embarrassed. I tried calling my mother and couldn't get her, and I cried.

I probably made five more trips to the bathroom while waiting for the doctor and went through half a roll of toilet paper. I was so nervous and kept wiping at every drop of blood. I was so embarassed, I was afraid I'd bleed through, even though I was barely bleeding. The amazing thing was that my younger sister, who I often think is a pain, really helped me out.

Finally, the doctor saw me, quickly figured out my "problem," and told my dad, who partially thought it was funny, partially was freaked out at such an obvious sign of my becoming a woman, and partially was pissed off for wasting our afternoon together at the hospital.

It was embarrassing at the time, but we laugh about it now. So as much as you are freaking, chances are once your period comes and becomes a natural part of your life, your first time will eventually become a funny story you share with your friends.

LAURA'S TIP: At first when you get your period, it seems like it's ruining your life. You fear the most normal things like going on a sleepover or on a date.

My mom said when she was younger some girls used to complain about their period (they called it their "friend") and cramps to get out of gym. I don't know anyone who does that anymore. A little period isn't going to stop me or my friends from living life to the fullest: sports, sleepovers, class trips, or whatever.

....

When I get my period, I get all moody and pick fights with my boyfriend for no reason. What's going on?

....

DR. MARLIN: Your body experiences changes in hormone levels, which may cause imbalances in brain chemicals such as seratonin that alter how you feel.

Doctors categorize menstrual changes as follows:

☀ Premenstrual changes: These include headache, fatigue, hunger, mood swings, and increased sensitivity to pain.
☀ Premenstrual syndrome (PMS): A number of the above symptoms happen together right around your period.
☀ Premenstrual disorder: These symptoms are so severe you can't function.
☀ Premenstrual exacerbate: Any chronic condition you already have gets worse just before your period. Alcoholics drink more, smokers smoke more, and bulimics binge and vomit more.

Around 25 percent of women have no emotional changes, 58 percent report moderate to severe symptoms, and about 7 percent suffer from true PMS.

If you have symptoms, keep track of them for a few months to see which category applies to you. Symptoms might include:

☀ Acne
☀ Backaches
☀ Fatigue
☀ Bloating
☀ Headaches
☀ Constipation
☀ Sore breasts
☀ Diarrhea
☀ Food cravings

Cutting down on chips and other salty foods will help with the bloating, since salt makes you retain water. PMS is usually at its worst the 7 days before your period starts, and it disappears when your period begins.

LAURA: When you're PMSing, warn the people most likely to come into your firing line (best friend, boyfriend, parents, siblings) that you're in a bad mood. Sometimes, just acknowledging the mood is enough to keep it in control. If you do find yourself losing it, use a control you've worked out in advance. I count to 10, find a room where I can be alone, put on my Walkman, and blast music.

While everyone around you will appreciate the effort, do it for yourself. The more you stay in control, the less damage control and guilt obsessing you'll have to do afterward.

Looking Your Best

When your body is rapidly changing, your feelings about how you look change as well. One study found that while 60 percent of elementary school girls considered themselves "happy the way I am," the number fell to a sad 29 percent by high school.

Turn on the TV, pick up a magazine, go to the movies, or walk by a billboard: You'd think skinny is the only kind of beautiful there is.

Everywhere there are images of perfect skin, perfect hair, perfect looks. Supermodel Cindy Crawford says, "People tell me women get upset because they don't look like this. What they don't realize is I *don't* look like this, either. They airbrush our every pimple, freckle, pore, and rounded chin."

How you look is important. But beauty is a state of mind as well as body. Low self-esteem and constant obsession over food and weight are not healthy, nor do they make you a fun person to be around.

· ·

How do you find a personal style? I always wear Levi's and a tee, which is boring. I love the way people like Madonna have a changing look.

· ·

LAURA'S TIP: My style evolved over the years. I used not to brush my hair and I wore black jumpsuits (it's a horror just to think about it now). As I got more interested in style, I bought more clothes and found things I liked. I tend to take something really fashionable but tone it down to suit me.

It helps to start small and change one thing at a time—maybe socks or nail polish color. This way you don't feel self-conscious and you slowly work out your new look.

Magazines show you fabulous clothes you're programmed to buy on fabulous models you're programmed to want to look like. The problem is that (a) you probably can't afford the clothes and (b) you're never going to be a supermodel.

It's better to read with a discerning eye and remember what fits your budget, taste, and needs. Cashmere, fur, and leather pants may be the rage for fall, but if you live in a warm climate you'll pass out from heat exhaustion while you break the bank to pay for them.

Trust your instincts and buy what appeals to your taste rather than what's on some editor's must-have list. If you can't afford the "real" thing, wait. Fashion is a cutthroat industry and you'll catch a knockoff soon.

....

I want to exercise, but I'm overweight and hate the looks I get, like "What's she trying to prove?"

....

DR. MARLIN: When you walk into a room, it's easy to imagine everyone is looking at you or thinking about you. Get some perspective. Chances are, you feel self-conscious because you are starting something new, not because you look odd.

Act as if there's no reason why you shouldn't be working out. Pretend you have a body you love and people will treat you the same way. If you stop judging yourself, others will pick up on your self-confident vibe and treat you with respect. They might see *you* instead of your nervousness.

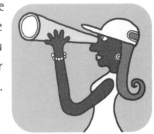

LAURA: When I would change in gym, I thought everyone was looking at me and judging the size of my breasts or thighs. But then I realized other girls were just as self-conscious about their bodies as I was. They were checking everyone else out because they felt weird about how *they* looked.

In the locker room the other day, everyone was complaining. I mean *everyone*. One girl said her nose is too big. Another kept talking about her thighs being huge. A third moaned that her legs are too short and her ankles too big. They all looked fine to me.

I remember in sixth grade everyone complaining about fat on some part of their body. I looked at them, then looked down, and figured that if their thighs were fat, mine were too, and I became very self-conscious about them. But the other day we pulled out some old videos and I wasn't fat at all! In fact, I was just the opposite. There was no reason for me to feel fat except for the fact that in comparison to these sticklike girls, I had meat on my bones. Not everyone looks like a model. Even models don't look like that. My friend's mother works for a magazine and we went through it and she pointed out how they had used the computer to make this one's stomach flatter and that one's boobs bigger.

If I asked my friends what they'd like to change about themselves, most

12 Things That Getting Fit Does for You (That Have Nothing to Do with Your Heart Rate)

1 Boosts self-esteem

2 Keeps you from getting fat

3 Makes you stand tall

4 Wipes out stress

5 Lifts depression

6 Makes you more likely to go to college

7 Makes you more optimistic

8 Gets you organized

9 Makes you less anxious

10 Helps you get focused

11 Channels your competitiveness in a positive way

12 Ups your GPA

Getting
Powerful

would say their weight, even though none of them are fat. No one would say she'd like to be more generous or patient or able. That's really sad. Maybe we all need to think like 8-year-olds again and just have fun and stop caring what we *think* other people think about us.

Eating Right

Eating right means listening to your body's internal signals (eating when you are hungry and stopping when you are full). But it is also knowing it's okay sometimes to eat for other reasons (the fresh cookies taste so good, or it will get you through an exam).

Studies show that 98 percent of those who lose weight by dieting not only gain it back but end up gaining more weight. When you starve yourself, your body slows down its metabolism to conserve calories. When you stop dieting, your body, which has been in starvation mode, reacts by storing any calories you give it as fat.

Dieting can make your nails brittle, your skin dry, your hair fall out, and your breath bad because you miss out on vital nutrients your body needs. You need nutrients and calories for energy when you work out (which is the healthiest way to control your weight, along with eating in moderation).

....

I take laxatives to keep my weight down. The box says you can take two a day for no more than a week. I've been taking two to six a day for two months. Is that dangerous?

....

DR. MARLIN: Yes, you are abusing them. Laxatives work by dehydrating you, which means they excrete the water and chemicals your body needs. Prolonged dehydration affects your entire gastrointestinal tract: Your intestines have trouble digesting food and your bowels stop working properly. The only way you can move your bowels is by taking more laxatives, which can lead to a dangerous cycle of addiction. And the loss of electrolytes through dehydration can affect your heart and kidneys.

It can be lethal, so you need to stop abusing these pills. If you stop abruptly, your body may react badly. Ask your doctor for a program to withdraw gradually, under his or her supervision.

LAURA: There are so many crazy ways that girls control their weight, from ipecac syrup to smoking, but taking laxatives is really gross. It causes gas and diarrhea. Imagine being out on a date when they kick in. The thing is, they don't even work. My doctor told me that diet pills only give the feeling of weight loss. By the time laxatives work, the calories have already been absorbed. You only feel like you've lost weight because you lost some water weight, which you'll regain in a few days. Big deal.

> I want to quit smoking, but I've heard that when you quit you gain weight. Is that true?

DR. MARLIN: Some people do, but a healthy person would have to gain almost 100 pounds in order to equal the health risks she gets with smoking.

If you eat the same as you did when you were smoking, your body will end up using less and storing more of the food as fat. Smoking also dulls the taste buds, so food begins to taste better when you stop smoking. And then there's oral fixation—some ex-smokers need something in their mouths to fill the void of cigarettes.

Low-calorie finger foods, such as carrot and celery sticks, will give you something to do with your fingers instead of holding a cigarette. Other things to put in your mouth include toothpicks, plastic straws, sugar-free gum, hard candy, and lollipops.

To reduce the craving to eat more, drink a glass of water before and during meals. Chew your food well, eat slowly, and enjoy how much better food tastes now. After a meal is a great time for a cigarette, right? Well, get up and move right away—wash the dishes, go for a walk, brush your teeth, eat a mint.

LAURA: I hate cigarettes, but lots of girls in my school do the cigarette diet. They don't lose weight, but they end up with smelly hair and clothes, bad breath, yellow teeth, and broke.

Am I Weird or Is This Normal?

Food Myths:
Separating the Fat from the Facts

MYTH: You can tell you need to lose weight by how you look.
FACT: Around 95 percent of women see themselves as 25 percent larger than they really are.

MYTH: You can tell you need to diet by how much you weigh.
FACT: Scales can't tell the difference between body fat and muscle, and we all know that muscle weighs more than fat.

MYTH: Dairy products are high in fat and should be avoided.
FACT: While you shouldn't gorge on them (low-fat alternatives are available), calcium is necessary for bone growth, especially in girls and young women.

MYTH: Vegetarians are healthier than meat eaters.
FACT: Diets that contain absolutely no animal products are very low in vitamin B_{12}, and, unless carefully

Eating Disorders

One out of every 10 teenage girls has an eating disorder.

Even though it's completely normal (and necessary) for girls to gain body fat during puberty, some girls respond by feeling compelled to get rid of it.

Some girls with eating disorders are depressed or have low self-esteem. Obsessively monitoring eating habits is a bad way to handle teenage stresses and anxieties.

Some sports can exacerbate a tendency to eating disorders. Gymnasts, ice skaters, runners, and ballerinas are told to lose weight. In planned, they may be deficient in vitamin B$_6$, riboflavin, calcium, iron, and zinc. Strict macrobiotic diets, which include everything except grains, are extremely hazardous.

MYTH: Since retinoic acid, a form of vitamin A, is often prescribed as a skin treatment for acne, a quicker way to cure acne is to swallow a lot of vitamin A supplements.

FACT: This could kill you. If you ingest too much vitamin A, you may suffer poisoning.

MYTH: Skipping breakfast is a good way to lose weight.

FACT: Breakfast is a must to get your blood sugar level up and give you energy you need to start the day. Otherwise, you'll crave sweets when energy levels dip around 11 A.M.

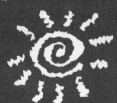

an effort to make their bodies smaller, leaner, faster, or stronger, these girls can end up with an eating disorder.

There is evidence that eating disorders tend to run in families. If a parent doesn't like her own body or is too concerned with her daughter's, it can increase the girl's chances for developing a disorder.

Whatever the cause, the effects can be devastating. As many as 20 percent of eating disorder patients starve themselves to death.

20 Really Gross Things
an Eating Disorder Does to You

1 You get toothaches and lose teeth.

2 Your breath gets bad.

3 You get lonely as you cut yourself off from friends and family to hide your secret.

4 Your friends stop calling you because they get bored with you obsessing about your weight all the time.

5 You can become blind (due to malnutrition).

6 You get vaginal dryness (which can make masturbation and/or sexual intercourse uncomfortable).

7 Your skin breaks out.

8 You stop doing things you enjoy because you lack the energy to do them.

9 Your legs and feet or your stomach get bloated.

10 You have problems falling and/or staying asleep.

11 You burp vomit (undigested food in your stomach).

12 You develop diabetes and have to inject insulin twice a day.

13 You lose interest in everything but your weight.

14 You get mood swings, alienating friends and family.

15 Your period stops.

16 You get cramps, constipation, diarrhea, and/or incontinence.

17 You look terrible.

18 Instead of feeling thin and in control of your life, you feel ashamed and like you want to die.

19 Once your eating disorder is known, you end up under 24-hour supervision.

20 You die.

Getting Powerful

···

My friend and I have gotten into this competitive thing to see who can eat the least amount
in a day. It's helping us lose weight, but I'm
scared we're making ourselves sick.

···

DR. MARLIN: Sometimes girls turn losing weight into a competition.
The result: What begins as mutual support becomes a group eating disorder. Get some perspective. The only good way to lose weight is to eat in
moderation and to exercise regularly. So instead of
starving yourselves together, sit down with your
friends and figure out a healthy plan along with
some fun workout things you can do together.

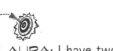

LAURA: I have two friends who take ballet together. They are always competing for the same
roles and they eat almost nothing, because each feels the other one will
get better parts if she weighs less. But even though both are disgustingly
thin, they seem to feel worse rather than better about themselves.

One Last Self-Acceptance Tip
from Dr. Marlin

Some of the changes during puberty are strange, uncomfortable,
even disgusting. But taking care of yourself helps you develop
healthy self-esteem so that you can like yourself for all the reasons
other people like you. Besides, your imperfections or inadequacies
do not define your value as a person. No one is confident about
everything at every moment.

When your body starts to change, it's easy to become obsessed
with what you think is wrong with the way you look. You compare
yourself to others unfavorably or let their opinions define you. So
you notice only your hips or breast size and not your soft skin or
strong hands or hearty laugh. You invest so much of your self-worth

in your appearance that it's almost impossible to feel good about yourself. Would you ever be half as harsh on someone else as you are on yourself?

Tell yourself you won't get what you want because you're fat and you probably won't. Not because you're fat but because you've given up. Convince yourself you'll blow everyone away at the play tryouts and the likelihood becomes greater that you will—that's called believing it.

Talk yourself into things, not out of them.

Getting Powerful

5
Getting Over It

Life is complicated. You feel incredibly confused, angry, and frustrated at times, then fine again without knowing why.

Such strong feelings come, in part, from the new hormones your body is producing. But there are other reasons.

You're having experiences for the first time: driving a car, working a part-time job, making decisions about schools, making choices about birth control.

You don't always know who to turn to for help. For example, your school teaches that alcohol is unhealthy and your parents say drinking is bad. But your friends say everyone is doing it and it feels good. However, you may feel out of control when you drink.

You're under similar pressure when it comes to deciding how to deal with sex, drugs, and who you want to be friends with. All this can make you unsure and nervous. But you can use your anxiety and turn it into resilience.

This chapter will help you get a handle on your emotions.

My parents have one image of me, my friends another, and my teachers yet another. No one gets the real me.

....

DR. MARLIN: You *are* different at different times with different people. But what defines you—your values and beliefs—stays the same.

Think of your personality as an orchestra: for example, the flutist, a little quiet but sweet; the violinist, shaky and high-pitched; the drummer, always wanting a solo; the brass, strident but strong. They all want to be heard. The conductor (your brain) has to make them play together.

There is no single "real you." You're the conductor of your own personal orchestra and the players are constantly changing. Sometimes you need more timpani, sometimes harp. They're all part of you.

LAURA: I don't know the "real me," either. My mother sees a sometimes moody, sometimes darling daughter, my father an alien young woman, my sister a pain in the ass, my best friend a fun and crazy pal, the boy next to me in homeroom a shy girl. Each sees only a part of me.

If I try to be the full me at one time, I'm weird. It's better to relax and just be who I am with each person. No one can know all of me. I just have to feel comfortable with all my selves.

Getting
Over It

....

One minute, I'm up and feel like I can do any-thing. A little later, everything sucks. I feel like I'm going crazy.

....

DR. MARLIN: Mood swings are a normal response to the stresses of being a teen. Some of them are linked to hormonal levels (see Chapter 4).

You may be short-tempered, touchy, down in the dumps, giddy, anxious, angry, or you may even feel like crying without knowing why. You may also be fine again without understanding what made you feel better.

Try to ride it out, because knowing you can have strong feelings without self-combusting is important. But if you find your emotions taking control—like you're yelling at your mother because she asked you to empty the dishwasher—then you need to put things in perspective or you may end up lower than before.

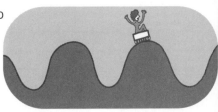

Self-exploration makes mood swings useful. Ask yourself:

★ What do I need to do to get over this?
★ What do I value enough to get upset about?
★ What do I crave?

And remind yourself: "This, too, shall pass."

LAURA: Once I was really upset for 2 days, I cried a lot, and I was mean for no good reason. Then, suddenly, I was laughing at a friend's joke and I felt fine. Once my mother told me I was behaving just like my neighbor's 2-year-old, and I knew exactly what she meant. When I babysit her, she'll sometimes cry hysterically for no other reason than she got dirt on her hands, and then she'll laugh hysterically because I gave her a toy to play with.

DR. MARLIN'S TIP: Watching television alone is one of the worst ways to relieve a bad mood because you just sit there instead of working it out. If you feel a bad mood coming on, reach out to your friends and yourself—go to an aerobics class, listen to music, call your favorite aunt.

· ·

It's difficult for me to concentrate on anything.

· ·

DR. MARLIN: You need to mellow out. Think about what you can change: Drop an activity? Switch your work hours? Reduce your class schedule?

Then try these simple stress busters when you feel tension:

1. Hold a pencil lightly by the point, letting the eraser hang straight down above a desk or table.

2. Rest your head against your other hand and close your eyes.
3. Slow your breathing and relax until the pencil slips naturally out of your fingers. Enjoy the calm for a few minutes.

Live in the moment. If you're doing dishes, push away all intruding thoughts. Instead, notice the warmth of the water, the smooth surface of the dish, the sensations of washing and rinsing. Use this stress reliever while walking, driving, shopping, cleaning, or working out.

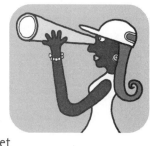

LAURA: I'm more stressed than anyone because I worry unnecessarily. I worry about grades, friends, life, everything. Just thinking about it now makes my heart beat fast. One way I cope—when I remember— is to get some perspective. I tell myself it's only high school—it's not life and death. My friends are my friends, even if I mess up once in a while. I also get someone to tell me everything's okay (my mom, a friend, a teacher), which makes me feel better. Oh, and my mom always tells me to breathe deeply, go for a run, or take a shower.

Getting
Over It

DR. MARLIN'S TIP: Don't wait for stress to get out of control. Here are some steps to stay on top of your life:

★ Don't procrastinate. Get things done as soon as you can. Say you finish your homework around 8 P.M. one night. Start working on any long-term projects that you have. Have an essay due next week? Do it now.

★ Be organized. Keeping a calendar lets you work more efficiently. After school, spend 10 minutes planning and writing down what the rest of your day will be like: 3–4 P.M.: rest and watch television; 4–5 P.M.: math homework; 5–7 P.M.: history project; 7–8 P.M.: dinner.

★ Know your limits. Activities are important for meeting new people and exploring new experiences, but you can overdo it. You could join the hockey team, write for the school newspaper, be president of your class, compete on the debate team. But chances are you can't do all of them. Focus on schoolwork first, then round out your schedule with extracurricular activities. One way to know if you're pushing yourself too far is if you feel that what you are about to do is a hassle or an intrusion on your time. This is the thing to drop.

....

I get so angry that I want to throw things and hit people. It scares me.

....

DR. MARLIN: You can't help how you feel, but you can control how you behave. The first step to ruling it is to give yourself distance from feeling angry and then doing something. Calling up a girlfriend to rehash the argument you just had with your boyfriend won't make you feel any better or more willing to work on the problem. It will just keep the fire of your anger burning.

Instead, give yourself time to decide how to handle the situation to your advantage. Ask yourself these questions:

★ Why am I angry? Be sure you're angry at one person or thing and not taking it out on someone else. For example, you may be angry at your teacher for giving you an unfair grade. But unable to confront your teacher, you go home and yell at your mother instead.

★ What do I want to accomplish? Revenge for being treated unfairly? Understanding? An apology? A compromise for a problem? Know what you want and let that guide you in how to express your feelings.

LAURA: It's so easy to get angry at everything. I have more responsibilities than ever—working, keeping my grades up to get into a good college, being an example to my younger sister, helping my mom around the house. And then there's the whole social scene, friends not being as great as I thought, wanting a boyfriend, and realizing good ones aren't easy to find. I can get very angry at times, and it takes all I have not to hit my sister or throw things. Sometimes I do throw things. I go into my room and fling pillows and scream. It sounds childish writing it, but I feel better getting it out of my system.

Feeling Sad and Bad

Psychiatric illnesses are disorders of the brain that disrupt a person's thinking, moods, and ability to relate to others. They do not make you a loser or a "crazy" person. They are not the result of personal weakness, lack of character, or poor upbringing. They are treatable. Many people need medication to help control symptoms. Supportive counseling and self-help groups can provide stability for recovery.

··

I feel like everyone is happy except me.

··

DR. MARLIN: People who describe themselves as happy have certain qualities in common, like the ability to make choices clearly and a knack for appreciating the good in their lives and taking responsibility for the bad. We all have it in our power to boost our happiness quotient.

Essentially, you need to rule it by making an attitude shift. First, quit complaining. Cold turkey. If you start to bitch, ask yourself what you can do about it. If your problem is an obnoxious so-called cool kid at school who makes your life hell, you can ignore her, tell her to shut up, or make a snappy comeback and then leave it. Taking action makes you feel good because it puts you in charge.

Also, decide every morning to have a great day. Set the alarm 10 minutes early and do something pleasant: Eat your favorite breakfast, read, write in your journal, or play with your pet. Use this time as your reminder signal to be happy. Then call up that happy feeling later when you fell crappy.

How to Stop Minimizing Yourself

During puberty, girls start to sprinkle their speech with such phrases as "I know this must sound stupid, but . . ." "It's not a big deal, but . . ." "I'm probably wrong, but . . ." They say they don't know things they actually do. They constantly worry about other people's reactions. And they doubt their right to speak up.

Here is how this works, in the words of a 27-year-old self-described apologizer:

A salesperson in a store tells me my backpack is unzipped and hanging open: "Oh, thank you, I'm sorry."

The urge is there all the time. Not only will I defer to a friend's choice of a movie, for instance, I feel bad and apologize if she insists we go to mine.

I apologize when I should simply say "thank you," because worry, guilt, and a need for reassurance seem to be part of everything I feel. It happens whenever my needs might possibly demand something of someone else. In other words, I apologize for being human.

I'm always uncomfortable on my birthday. I want to be loved and appreciated, but I worry about people taking the time and trouble to show they care about me.

I even apologize for apologizing too much. My everyday speech is filled with words and phrases such as, "anyway," "just," and "I don't know" to disclaim what I'm going to say and apologize in advance for wasting the

LAURA: A friend of mine who seemed to have a perfect life went into a severe depression. She said, "I had everything I ever wanted and I still wasn't happy." That made me realize that a cute guy or lots of friends or *listener's time. What complicates all this is a nagging awareness that my behavior can be irritating and unattractive. I feel like a stereotype of our culture's stupid standard of femininity for girls and young women (assertive, demanding, and unyielding is "bad," gracious, diminutive, and deferential is "good"), and I'm angry that I've internalized that message.*

I need to remember that there is a huge difference between being thoughtful and apologizing for your existence.

After all, I love going to my friends' birthday parties. I love celebrating them, supporting them, and listening to them, even when they ramble. Sometimes most of all when they ramble.

Essentially, learning to stop apologizing all the time means learning to accept that you are, in fact, only human. And to be human is to have needs, make mistakes, lose control, and fall short of pleasing every single human being on the planet every minute. Speaking up is the best thing you can do for yourself.

While self-effacing behavior can feel safe and even be charming, putting yourself down all the time is just as damaging as if someone else were putting you down all the time. Despite the messages the media may send us, people like to be around self-assured, confident women. The grand apologizer is a turnoff.

a 4.0 GPA doesn't guarantee happiness. So when I am feeling really down, I try to get some perspective by realizing others out there feel as low as I do. It's a bonding of sorts and makes me feel better.

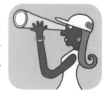

Avoid These Four Downers

1 Drugs: Mind-altering substances get results right away. But once the buzz is gone, so is the good mood, and you feel worse.

2 Sugar snacking: Sweets may give you an initial boost of energy, but in an hour you feel even more sluggish, tense, and irritable. Then you crave another sugar fix.

3 TV: If you zone out to avoid unpleasant moods, you are likely to feel tired, drained, and guilty after you hit the off button. It's hard to pick yourself up off the couch and deal with feelings you were avoiding.

4 Driving: It's tempting but not wise to put your foot on the gas and escape to the highway. In a bad mood you are less likely to focus on the rules of the road.

I have no energy or interest in anything anymore. I just want to stay in bed.

DR. MARLIN: If you feel lethargic and out of it for a while, you may be clinically depressed. Common causes include family tension, school stress, and traumatic events (such as parents divorcing, a death of someone close to you, breaking up with a boyfriend). So if you don't understand exactly why you've been down and it's lasted more than a few days, view your feelings as warnings. Depression isn't always marked by sadness and crying.

If you ignore or deny your feelings, your depression may come out in destructive ways: a drop in grades, boredom, ditching school, experimenting with drugs, violence, impulsiveness, obsessive thoughts, and/or eating disorders.

LAURA: Sometimes I think you just have to give in to your sad feelings and see where they take you. There are times when I've felt tired, irritated, and sad and sat around the house watching TV in my purple pajama bottoms. My mother hates them, because she knows what they mean and she's not a believer in the TV as a pick-me-up. But by the end of the day, I am so bored that I begin to appreciate my friends and don't even mind my little sister bugging me.

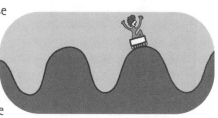

. . . .

I sometimes think about killing myself. I don't want to have these thoughts, but I do.

. . . .

DR. MARLIN: Lots of people are walking around with thoughts like yours. But most don't act on them (see "10 Suicide Warning Signs" on page 158 to assess your risk level).

You may have these thoughts:

Getting
Over It

★ "I'm a total failure."
★ "Everyone hates me."
★ "My parents don't get me."
★ "People will finally pay attention if I kill myself."

Sometimes the worst part of these thoughts is how shameful they are. Sharing them with a trusted person, such as a therapist, can help immeasurably. Speaking with a family member, a teacher you like, a school counselor, or a friend's parent could also help. If you ever find your thoughts unbearable, 24-hour anonymous hot lines can provide immediate assistance and referrals in your area (see "Address Book" on page 255).

LAURA: I've thought about killing myself mainly in a "They'll be sorry when I'm gone" way. I'm sure every other kid my age has had such

10 Bad-Mood Busters

1 Think positive. When you have a depressing thought, such as "I can't do Latin," substitute, "With the right help, I can do Latin" and seek out a teacher, tutor, or friend.

2 Keep a good news journal and make yourself write in it before going to bed; you don't write the bad stuff here, only good things that happened during the day. It may not be easy at first, but include items like a stranger smiled at you. If you do this faithfully, it keys your mind to look for the positive. Studies show suicidal people getting better after just two weeks of doing the good news journal.

3 Spend time with anyone who makes you laugh.

4 Pay attention to when you feel what you feel. Mood awareness can help you match tasks with your energy levels: If you're at your best in the morning, for instance, that's the time to deal with stressful chores, like confronting a friend who hurt you or talking to a teacher who you feel misgraded you. If you routinely feel drained in the late afternoon, reserve those hours for activities that don't require much emotional energy: Catch up on your reading or spend time with

thoughts. Or fantasized about killing that snotty little bitch who's always making snide remarks about you. But thinking about the reality—how sad and hurt my family would be, how much I really don't hate my life enough to end it—stops me from doing anything.

friends. Never undertake anything stressful when you're tired or tense.

5 Observe your moods at different times of the month. Some women find bad moods coincide with their menstrual cycle (see Chapter 4).

6 Exercise keeps you fit mentally as well as physically. As little as 20 minutes daily can bring a sense of calm and well-being. This will boost your body's production of endorphins—chemicals we all have that create a natural high.

7 Get some perspective.

8 Listen to music. One study found that rhythm provides structure and security and helps to reduce muscle tension.

9 Call your friends. Reaching out makes you feel connected and less isolated. And getting hugged can release feel-good hormones to help you cope.

10 Surround yourself with happy people. Moods are highly contagious. We unconsciously imitate facial expressions, muscular movement, posture, and speech patterns to match those we are with.

Getting
Over It

LAURA'S TIP: If you have a friend contemplating suicide, let someone know. Trust is one of the major building blocks of friendship, but absolute secrecy goes out the window when a friend is in danger. If you're scared she's going to hurt herself, tell a trustworthy adult.

10 Suicide Warning Signs

1. Withdrawal from friends or family and no desire to go out
2. Inability to concentrate or think clearly
3. Change in eating or sleeping habits
4. Major changes in appearance (if a normally neat person looks very sloppy, for example)
5. Talk about feeling hopeless or feeling guilty
6. Talk about suicide
7. Talk about death
8. No desire to take part in favorite activities
9. Giving away favorite possessions (if someone offers you his or her favorite piece of jewelry, for example)
10. Suddenly very happy and cheerful moods after being depressed or sad for a long time (someone who has decided to attempt suicide may feel it's a "solution")

If you or a friend experiences any of these signs, see "Address Book" on page 255 for help.

Losing Control with Drugs

Only you can decide whether you abstain from drugs totally, or try everything, but remember that whether you experiment or become a regular user, you are at a high risk for becoming addicted. Since your main raison d'être right now is breaking free and living for yourself, why blow that independence by getting hooked on a drug? Know what you're getting into. Get yourself educated about the real facts of life when it comes to drugs, so that you can be in control when you want to be, and not be controlled by others (your folks, your friends, the drugs) when you don't want to be.

Getting Help

Historically there has been a stigma attached to seeing a therapist; some people are still embarrassed or ashamed. But mental health problems are just like physical problems—in fact, we're discovering that some mental illnesses have chemical and/or biological causes, or are intensified by physical conditions.

Getting help is a sign of strength, not weakness. It's a sign of courage. In fact, it's more courageous than hiding behind a mask of false well-being if you're hurting inside.

When you talk to your parents about a touchy subject—like doing drugs or having sex—they sometimes automatically assume that if you are asking about it, you are doing it. Going to a guidance counselor, school psychologist, or other therapist gives you a safe place to put issues like these on the table, to explore and figure out your options with an adult without worrying about being yelled at, ridiculed, or hurting someone's feelings.

It doesn't have to take years. For instance, cognitive-behavioral therapy deals with specific problems in your life right now—such as the breakup of a relationship, fear of independence—rather than what has gone on in the past. You learn effective ways of coping with your feelings and changing your behavior. Try your school counselor. You can find a therapist through school (teacher, nurse, or counselor), trusted friends, your doctor, clergy, or your family. There are groups, free clinics, private practice, family therapy, and low-cost clinics at hospitals.

Getting
Over It

Eight Reasons People Get High (And What to Do Instead)

Understanding why some people use drugs can help you make a decision about what you want to do:

1 Curiosity: Some people want to know how drugs will make them feel. Instead, do some adrenaline-rush activity you've never done before but always wanted to try—like snowboarding.

2 False confidence: Drugs make you lose control of your inhibitions. This is not the same as having confidence. If you become dependent on drugs, that saps your confidence. Try out for the school play. Actors use a persona to show confidence they may not have in real life.

3 To feel good: Initially, drugs may induce euphoria. But to maintain that, you will have to take more and more drugs to get the same feeling. Go to a comedy club. Laughter is a quicker and safer route to feeling euphoric.

I don't really want to do drugs, but when I'm at a party and other kids are getting high, I feel pressured to join in.

DR. MARLIN: As I constantly tell Laura, stop thinking either-or. You don't have to choose to *either* go along with the group *or* be your own person. Do both. Being yourself doesn't preclude being part of a group any more than being part of a group means you can't think for yourself.

Arm yourself with information about what drugs do and what they keep you from doing. You don't have to share that information with anyone else. You don't want to seem like a know-it-all or a nag. But knowing

4 To get attention: Sometimes taking drugs is a cry for help—an attempt to get parents, friends, and the world at large to notice to your pain. Talk to an ally about your pain.

5 Peer pressure: You don't want to feel left out or made fun of if your friends are taking drugs. Find true friends who will respect your standing up for your convictions.

6 Social status: You may think taking drugs will make you cool. Doing your own thing makes you cool.

7 To escape: Drugs can be a way of numbing you from dealing with the problems in your life. Listen to music to get your mind off your problems. It will leave you with the energy to deal with them. Prayer has the same effect.

8 To rebel: Drugs are illegal and therefore doing them can make you feel more grown up. There are better and more effective ways to rebel (see Chapter 7).

Getting Over It

that heroin is addictive even if smoked and that trying coke once can kill you will remind you of why you don't want to do drugs.

People who put pressure on you aren't real friends. Friends look out for your best interests and respect you when you don't want to do what they do.

LAURA: Lots of kids in my school manage to smoke weed and still get straight A's, be stars on varsity sports teams, and be anything but the stereotypical burnout. But it's not something that interests me. I am included and invited to things—no one calls me a dork.

The truth is that doing all that stuff is not what makes you cool—it's how you act about it. If you just say no and act like it's no big deal and don't get all nervous, then it's no big deal.

LAURA'S TIP: If you feel pressured to do stuff you don't want to do, maybe you should think about finding a new group. Not because they do drugs, but because they seem so desperately to want you to do drugs.

....

My friends and I get high a lot on the weekends. I'd like to stop, but I always get bored when I'm not stoned.

....

DR. MARLIN: To break the cycle, do things that you couldn't do if you were high—play a sport, take a long drive, volunteer, climb a tree. All of these require sharp, clear-minded concentration. Learning "natural high"

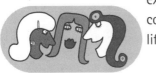

exercises like yoga or meditation can help you cope with stress that'll come from changing your lifestyle.

The longer you take the drugs, the harder it will be to stop—that's how addiction works.

LAURA: Doing the same thing over and over again can get boring no matter if it's getting high or going to the mall. Sitting around doing nothing can be boring, and if that's what you're doing when you're high and when you're not, of course it will be more interesting when you're high. But get off your ass and get high naturally—you'll lift your mood, get more energy, and be less likely to look for artificial ways to relieve your boredom.

Laura's Top 10 Favorite Natural Highs

1 Make someone laugh.

2 Run around the block.

3 Have an orgasm.

4 Fly a kite.

5 Sing out loud at the top of your voice.

6 Lie in bed listening to the rain outside.

7 Take a bubble bath.

8 Run through sprinklers.

9 Make eye contact with a cute stranger.

10 Hug someone you love.

Getting
Over It

Four High Downers

1 Driving and taking drugs (including alcohol): Every 23 minutes someone dies because of a drunk driver.

2 Becoming permanently disabled or dying: Many drugs, such as LSD, speed, and heroin, can cause permanent psychosis and even death on the first try. In addition, the purity of drugs available has more than quadrupled, making it easier to become addicted or to overdose.

3 Making big decisions about sex while under the influence (see Chapter 3).

4 Mixing alcohol with other drugs—even legal ones: For instance, if you take a cold pill and then go out drinking, you're combining two depressants, which can kill you. The same goes if you combine a downer with alcohol. And if you're taking an antibiotic and drinking, the antibiotic may be inactivated.

I've only smoked the occasional joint and sometimes drink beer. But my parents are convinced that I'm going to be a druggie. They constantly watch me and go through my things. Now they're threatening to give me a drug test. How can I get them to lay off?

DR. MARLIN: Here's how parents think: You've done drugs. You've been drinking. Therefore, it's a short hop and skip to "my daughter the druggie alcoholic." One poll found that three times as many parents worry about their teens getting involved with drugs and alcohol than their children themselves do. Obviously, there's a gap in concerns here.

Is their behavior an overreaction? Probably. But the goal isn't to control you; it's to keep you safe. Your parents feel it's their job to keep you from making mistakes. So here's how to get them to back off: Keep them informed. This way, they'll get an idea of what's going on in your life, but it will be on your terms.

LAURA: I feel like I am told not to have sex, not to smoke, not to drink, not to let others pressure me into doing things. I don't think that I have gone out once when my mother hasn't warned me not to drink or do drugs (always with some stupid reason, too, like you're on cold medicine and you'll get sicker if you do anything bad).

I don't want to live by my parents' and teachers' expectations. I want to live the way I want to. I don't want to be protected from making mistakes. If I don't make mistakes, I will never learn.

But I've also learned from experience that the only way to get my mother off my back is to not just tell her but show her I am being responsible and smart about my life. I notice she backs off more when I make sure my grades are good and pay attention to her curfews than when I just try and argue her out of her position.

Alcohol

Although it is illegal for anyone under the age of 21 to purchase, possess, and/or consume alcohol, nearly half of all Americans over the age of 12 consume alcohol.

> My father is an alcoholic and I'm scared I may go the same way. Whenever I drink, I don't seem to be able to stop.

DR. MARLIN: Alcoholism is genetic, so it is possible that you have inherited your father's addiction. Children of alcoholics are about four times more likely to become alcoholic than others.

Alcoholism develops in stages, beginning with a preoccupation with

Women and Alcohol

Women have a lower tolerance for alcohol than men. Within minutes of drinking the same amount of alcohol as a man, your blood alcohol level may be 25 to 30 percent higher. The difference is only partly due to the fact that most women are smaller than men and therefore their bodies absorb alcohol more quickly.

Another key factor is that the enzyme that metabolizes alcohol in the stomach is less active in women than men. So more alcohol goes directly into your bloodstream and gets there more quickly.

All this means you not only get intoxicated faster, but you're more likely to have liver damage from excessive drinking. Drinking also makes you less likely to be in control.

Blood alcohol concentration (BAC) is the amount of alcohol in the bloodstream. It is measured in percentages. For instance, having a BAC of 0.10 percent means that a person

drinking and advancing to complete physical dependence. Not being able to control your drinking is certainly one symptom of the disease.

In your case it's asking for trouble to continue drinking. If you're scared you may go the same way as your dad, use your fear. Ask yourself why you drink: to fit in, out of habit, or boredom? No answer could be sufficient to compete with your terror of becoming an alcoholic.

And it doesn't matter what you drink. Wine is typically 8 to 14 percent alcohol, whereas beer is 4 to 6 percent "firewater" by volume. However, while hard liquor looks as though it has more alcohol by volume, the larger serving sizes of wine and beer make it very easy to drink the same amount of alcohol, if not more. (Light beer isn't really lighter in the alcohol department than regular beer; it just has fewer calories.) So a "drink" is considered any alhas 1 part alcohol per 1,000 parts blood in the body. When your BAC is 0.02 percent (substantially below the 0.10 percent legal standard in most states for drunkenness), your motor skills, ability to react to a crisis, vision, concentration, and understanding and perception of a potentially dangerous situation—like rape—are all affected. In addition, studies have found that 25 to 50 percent of non-fatal intentional injuries involve alcohol, including rape. However, these stats may also include the rapist. Also, according to law enforcers, drunkenness at the time of a rape affects the victim's ability to describe the exact sequence of events, and that makes her a target for the defense. Even when a rape victim can clearly recall what happened, her drinking may make the jury less sympathetic. A Pennsylvania State University study suggests that rapists are generally held less accountable for attacks if they're drunk; intoxicated victims are held more accountable.

coholic beverage that contains half an ounce of pure ethanol. That usually translates into either 5 ounces of wine (average glass), 12 ounces of a wine cooler (average serving), 12 ounces of beer (average serving), or 1.5 ounces (average serving) of 80 proof distilled liquor, such as whiskey, scotch, rum, or vodka.

LAURA: I know at least three kids whose parents are alcoholics and it's scary to watch them going the same way. One started off saying she was never going to drink because her mom is drunk all the time. Then she was out on a date and the guy she was with pressured her. Now she comes to school drunk sometimes. Another used to drink only at parties, but now he drinks when he's just hanging with his friends. The other girl said she was only going to drink beer, which she still does. And now she drinks a six-pack a day.

Did You Know Alcohol . . .

1 Lowers sex drive

2 Makes you more likely to have unprotected sex

3 Gives you bad breath

4 Makes you fat (the calories from alcohol are stored in your fat cells)

5 Makes you violent (even at low doses it has been shown to increase aggressive behavior—half of homicides involve alcohol, as do one-quarter to one-third of suicides)

6 Makes you feel sick (some people get hangovers—headache, nausea, thirst, dizziness, and fatigue)

7 Puts you at risk of being raped (you're vulnerable)

Smoking

Every day about 3,000 teens start smoking. At least one-third will die early as a result. Those who start smoking before age 21 have the hardest time breaking the habit.

What's the big deal if I just smoke one cigarette a week?

DR. MARLIN: Because chances are you'll change your habit—for the worse. Young people who list themselves as "occasional smokers" end up being at least pack-a-day smokers by the time they are 20. Not only that—smoking actually *increases* anxiety.

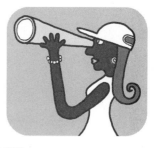

Cigarettes are made with nicotine, a substance as addictive as heroin. One-third of all smokers make serious attempts to quit each year, but 80 percent of them resume their habit within 12 months. Even if you manage to quit, your craving can last for days, months, years, or a lifetime.

LAURA: Lots of my friends who smoke a pack a day started with the "just one-a-day" route. It doesn't work.

Tobacco companies want to get teens hooked on smoking because they need to recruit 1,200 new smokers every day to replace those who die. Ads show gorgeous guys and girls deliriously happy as they do outdoorsy things, kiss, and dance around. The models are all skinny to make us think cigarettes will stop us from gaining weight. Tobacco companies want us to think that if we smoke we'll have the perfect life (instead of bad breath, yellow teeth, wrinkled skin, and health problems). Think about that the next time you light up. Gross.

One Last Survival Tip from Dr. Marlin

The traits for a survivor personality are a lot like muscles—they need to be developed. And if you stop using them, they get weak.

True survivors find some way to seize control, even in desperate situations. Consider a 17-year-old patient of mine who was beaten, raped, and thrown into the trunk of a car. She found the wires to the tail lights and ripped them out. When the police pulled the driver over, she screamed and saved her life. The next time you're up against a wall, think about what you can do to affect the outcome.

People who can see the glass half full in life are likely to survive big blows. They put on a positive spin without wallowing in self-blame when things go wrong. Suppose someone fails an exam, gets in a car accident, or gets dumped by a boyfriend. The pessimist will

Kick Ash

Smoking is addictive (some tobacco companies manipulate tobacco to increase the brain's absorption of nicotine) and you may need help to stop. Here are ways to kick the habit:

★ List your reasons for wanting to quit. Read them every day.
★ Set a quit date and tell people about it.
★ Throw away all cigarettes, lighters, and matches.
★ Join a stop-smoking group (see "Address Book" on page 255).
★ Avoid other smokers while you're quitting.
★ Identify danger times for you such as a meal or at a party (keep a journal for at least 3 days— 1 school day and the weekend—about where and when you tend to smoke most often). This will stop you from mindlessly lighting up.
★ Eat three meals a day to keep your blood sugar up, which will reduce your urge to smoke.
★ Ask your doctor to prescribe nicotine patches.
★ See an acupuncturist for quit-smoking treatments.
★ When you want to smoke, have substitutes like licorice sticks or carrots ready.
★ Reward yourself and keep adding to your list of benefits of quitting.

say, "I'm a loser and my life sucks." The optimist will say, "I made a mistake, but the trouble is only temporary."

Learning from your past actions builds your survival skills. Look back on a stressful episode and consider how you could have handled it better. Mentally rehearse doing it a different way. For example, if you were with friends who were shoplifting and you were scared, think about what you could have done: left when you realized what was going on and told them you'd see them later, or not gone in the first place because you know this is what they do at the mall.

Make sure replaying the past doesn't turn into a bout of brooding or blaming yourself. Feeling guilty can be a way of avoiding change: You take the blame and think that's all you have to do. You are doing this if you find yourself saying "I'm sorry" constantly. Instead, think of what you've done that can make you say, "I'm proud."

Getting
Over It

6
Getting Cool

Friends are as important as food, water, and breathing. Sometimes more. Which is why it's so vital to choose people who you feel a true kinship with (you enjoy their company, you feel you can be yourself around them, and you know that they will support and sustain you without judgment).

Making Friends

It doesn't matter how many people you count as your nearest and dearest in your buddy list. You should never stop reaching out and making friends. Why?

For one thing, one person can't possibly fulfill all the needs of another. So not only will a broader circle of friends give you more to share with the friends you already have, but it will mean you always have someone to hang with.

People always think I'm bitchy and stuck-up, but actually I'm shy. How can I make them see the real me?

DR. MARLIN: You have lots of company. Nearly 50 percent of people are shy (see Chapter 5). The majority have figured out how to hide their ill-at-ease feelings. But they still suffer internally. Many people seem to be born shy; others develop shyness later in life.

Unfortunately, when you're shy it's easy to give the wrong impression that you're cold, indifferent, or a snob because you keep your head down, don't talk, and forget to smile.

The fact is your shyness is never going to completely disappear. But you can control it and lessen its effect on you by knowing your strengths.

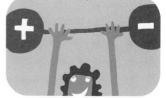

LAURA: I know how hard it is—it took me about 10 years to get over my shyness. Here's what I found helped me:

- ◉ I try to keep track of any compliments I get and repeat them to myself. It doesn't convince me I'm great, but it gives me a boost when I need it and *that* makes me feel less shy.
- ◉ It took me a while to realize this, but no one expects you to talk like Chandler on *Friends* all the time. You can say dumb stuff and not have everyone laugh at you.
- ◉ Skip the saying hi to everyone because it isn't that easy to do if it isn't in your nature. Instead, look for other people like you— really nice on the inside and waiting for someone to realize it. And they will be happy (and grateful) to connect.
- ◉ Target a couple of the more outgoing kids in school and ask them about some upcoming event. Don't become their shadow or they'll get pissed. But just talking to them a couple of times a week will probably get them to start saying hi to you and make you seem less bitchy to other people.

DR. MARLIN'S TIP: Here are eight tips I suggest to my patients who want to get a grip on shyness. At least one is bound to work for you:

Getting Cool

1. *Go on-line.* When you're cyber-talking, you can be anyone you want to be. This gives you the opportunity to try on different personalities and even audition jokes and topics before trying them out for real.

   Never plan a face2face. Chat rooms can be a great way to meet people in virtual reality, but it is never a good idea to take it a step closer to real life. You just don't know who you're talking to.

   Also, never give out any personal info on-line, like your full name, where you live, what school you go to, what your phone number is, credit card numbers, and so on. The reason? You don't want anyone infiltrating your life in case they turn out to be dangerous.

2. *Use people's names when speaking to them.*

3. *Ask questions or seek clarification (even if you really do understand what the person means).* This will give you instant conversation material, but be careful not to come across as someone who isn't listening.

4. *Join in existing conversations rather than trying to initiate one.* If your voice is shaky, make brief comments.

5. *Give compliments.* This is a one-per-customer deal, since over-praising makes you seem phony. But if you're talking to someone and don't know what to say, offer up a compliment (you can always find something nice to say—you like their manicure, T-shirt, whatever). Everyone loves flattery. It makes other people feel good and glad they talked to you.

6. *Carry a prop.* It's natural when you're shy to want to cross your arms, which screams, "Keep out!" Instead, put one hand in your pocket, on your hip, or over the arm of a chair. If necessary, hold a pen or a can of soda—anything to keep your arms unfolded.

7. *Unfocus.* If you just can't look the other person in the eye, focus on the "third" eye—the space precisely between the eyebrows. You'll appear to be making direct eye contact.

8. *Volunteer.* Do something to help others. Offer to serve the drinks at a party or tutor younger kids. Helping others will give you something to do, and that makes you feel like you belong because you have a reason for being there. And the more you join

activities that interest you, the more you will place yourself in situations where you have to talk to people—the bonus is that the activity gives you something to talk about.

My family just moved to a new state and I hate it. I don't know anyone, and everyone at school seems so tight that I don't see how I can ever penetrate their circles.

DR. MARLIN: Moving is not a transition anybody makes quickly. The usual adjustment is about 6 months, so give yourself time. Instead of wallowing at home alone, try flipping your thinking and riding it out.

Yes, it's hard to start over, but it can also be fun. You're entering a time in life when you might want to bury some of the things from your past and start new. Just think—you can reinvent yourself.

The more things you get involved in, the more people you are going to meet who are interested in the same things you like—always a good conversation starter. There are always groups and clubs that need people. You can make the best friends when you share an interest with them.

I'm not saying you should totally change your personality. Or even that it will be easy. But getting involved will help you to blend in rather than just standing around and being the new girl everyone stares at.

LAURA: All you really need is to meet one person. Then you'll meet that person's friends and things will happen naturally.

Here's what helped me when I switched to a school where I didn't know anyone:

◎ I pretended to myself that I had been the most popular person in my old school. This gave me the confidence to approach people and talk to them.

⚬ I called my best friend daily and got all my whining done with her. This kept me from off-loading on the first person who smiled at me.

⚬ I looked for people who dressed like me rather than those who dressed the coolest. I thought if we look alike, we might have something in common.

⚬ I joined the tennis team. I'm not that good, but I love playing. So I figured I might find a partner to play with.

⚬ When someone gave me their phone number, I used it. I called and asked about homework or if they knew a cool place to hang out. This was really hard because there was a chance they were just doing it to be polite. But if they blew me off, at least it wouldn't be in person. Also, calling meant they couldn't see my red face and sweaty hands. I practiced what I was going to say before I called and kept it short—the point was just to make contact.

The In-Crowd

We feel that our friends represent who we are. But how popular you were in high school is definitely not important for your future. *Popular* barely even exists in the same context in college, where there are so many people that no one thinks about who is coolest or best.

In fact, it seems your chances of being cool later in life are inversely related to your popularity level in school (okay, we have no hard data on this, but if you go by interviews made by many celebrities, they were all nerds in school; for instance, Winona Ryder, Keanu Reeves, Thurston Moore, Ice-T, Veronica Webb, Bill Gates . . . get the picture?). Think about it this way: If your best moments in life occur in tenth grade, isn't it going to be all downhill from there?

Still, you're dealing with high school, where coolness is definitely power-packed with meaning, so let's get on with it.

....

I don't feel like everyone else and don't want to be some conformist, but at the same time I'm scared of sticking out.

....

DR. MARLIN: Of course, you want to be unique. And, of course, you don't want to be an outsider. That can be very lonely. You can manage both by taking some risks—*slowly.* Think of it as trying to balance yourself in the middle of a seesaw.

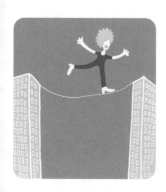

Start breaking out when you're with close friends or anyone you feel comfortable with who you know won't cold-shoulder you for being different from them.

The big fear is that you'll seem strange. But weird can be dreaded (being the outcast who's just too different) or the highest compliment.

You'll discover that as frightening as it is to stand out from the crowd, it can also be liberating to make this sort of impact. Among all the other separate selves out there in the world, you are now a force in your own right: a genuine and unshrinking "me" in a mass of others.

The point is that you don't have to dye your hair purple to stand out. You can be different just by being yourself and finding other people who are also comfortable with sticking out.

Getting Cool

LAURA: I always wanted to be my own person, but it just seemed too scary. Look at the kids who pierce their eyebrows, play the bagpipes, dress really conservatively—I knew this one kid who became a Hare Krishna practically overnight. These kids get labeled weird for doing their own thing. So I usually just went with the crowd and hated it. I'd write countless pages in my journal about how I felt.

Part of my problem was that I could never figure out *how* I wanted to be different or who I really was. I thought I had to be like one of those weird kids and do something dramatically different to stand out. But that's not me, either. That's why it's really hard to do your own thing.

What I realized about myself is that I didn't really want people to notice me. I just wanted to be able to do things because I liked them and not because everyone else was doing them—like go to the movies I wanted to see and wear clothes that I wanted to wear and get involved in activities that interested me. So what I do isn't so major in that I stand out, but it makes me feel more comfortable with who I am.

Also, don't be so close-minded about the "normal" stuff; if you like the new color that everyone is wearing, it's okay to wear it without automatically conforming.

DR. MARLIN'S TIP: Your identity is influenced by at least three things:

1. The genes you inherit from your family spark your artistic talent or your science skills and also influence your personality, including whether you're shy or outgoing, fast-paced, or relaxed, and so on.
2. Your cultural background influences your identity through the beliefs, language, customs, religion, and values taught to you by your family.
3. Your environment—your friends, school, neighborhood, and the media—also contribute to who you are.

One way to stand out is to start thinking about which of the above are your main influences. Here are some questions to answer in your journal to spark your thinking about your identity:

- What quality most defines your friends?
- What about your boyfriends and crushes?
- If you could come up with one thing you'd like people to remember you for, what would it be and why?
- Name five things you like about yourself. Name five things you wish you could change.
- What has been the happiest moment in your life? Why?
- Who has most influenced your life? Why?
- What has been your most embarrassing moment? Why?
- When you have a problem, is your first reaction to think it over or to immediately do something about it?

- ◉ What is your favorite place?
- ◉ What is your most important goal right now?

Now write a paragraph starting with "I am" that includes all of the above answers. This is your key to who you are and what is most important to you.

Dealing with Prejudice

You can't change someone's racist beliefs overnight. But here's what you can do immediately:

- ◉ Start with yourself. Acknowledge that you are different. Say it to yourself over and over if you have to. Yes, it's hard. But you can't change it. Embracing your background rather than fighting it will make you feel less like a victim.

  Get involved and find out what your ethnic background and cultural identity mean. For example, if you're African-American, learn about the black experience in America. If you're disabled, know your rights. If you're gay, find out about the gay movement and gay pride.

  You might reach out to others with similar backgrounds and needs both within and outside your community. Also, someone with similar life experiences is only a click away on the Internet, or if you don't have Internet access and can't get it through your school or library, you can try finding a pen pal.

- ◉ Speak up when you've been offended by a racial joke or another expression of racism, even if you're not a member of the group that has been attacked. All too often the party that has been offended is left with the responsibility of pointing out a slight, which should be recognized by everyone.

  But don't attack personally by saying something like, "How can you say that?" It'll only make the person who

Getting Cool

made the remark defensive and unwilling to discuss it. Instead, counter the derogatory remark with a positive one.

⊚ Also be willing to acknowledge your own prejudices and fears. Ask yourself how many of your friends come from backgrounds different from your own. Ask yourself why you may feel uncomfortable around people of different races. Are you ignorant of their beliefs and customs? Are you afraid you'll say or do the wrong thing? Do you think they don't want to get to know you?

Best Friends

People undergo so many changes—both physically and mentally—that it can affect your relationships with them. You change at different rates, develop new interests, want to get in with certain cliques—all these changes present new challenges. Even a friend who you've always agreed with might suddenly disagree with you on something important.

My best friend, another friend, and I have always been super close. But now the two of them leave me out. They never call and when I invite them over they make up excuses. Why are they locking me out?

DR. MARLIN: I can't think of many things that are as painful as being dumped out of the blue by your friends. The thing to remember is that your friends' cruelty probably has nothing to do with you. Chances are they're feeling insecure, and ganging up on you is a temporary and false confidence booster. Pathetic, yes—but all too common.

Here's what to do if you want to keep the friendships: Try to get each one alone and say that you're feeling hurt and alienated and still want to be friends (together they will pretend that they don't know what you are talking about and you'll just be giving them one more thing to bond over).

But maybe you should go the other route and reach out and make some new friends—people who share your interests and will include you in their plans because they want to.

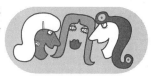

LAURA: My math teacher says the thing about odd numbers (like three) is that they don't divide evenly.

The good news is this practice of exiling people to social Siberia is very high school. It eases up as you get older and the best-friendship stakes become less intense.

DR. MARLIN'S TIP: Three-way friendships don't always have to be about backstabs and betrayals. For one thing, they take the sting out of the natural competition that exists between friends.

They ease the 24-hour responsibility that goes along with being a good friend. And they break up the intensity of a twosome, where a certain dress alike–talk alike–think alike twinishness can pervade. In a triangle, if you aren't alike, you split your differences; for instance, one friend may be the talker, another the thinker, and the third the doer.

But a lot of times the connection balance shifts. It could be that right now your friends have more in common with each other than with you; for example, they both play defense on the basketball team or like horror movies. So they might be closer to each other now, but by year's end the balance may have shifted and you'll have more in common with one of them.

Getting Cool

Which isn't much help to you right now, I know. But it might help you get some perspective about waiting around for one of them to call you.

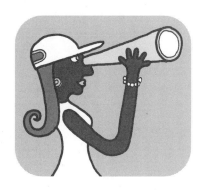

• •

I found out that my friends had a sleepover and didn't invite me. Why would they do that? I feel so hurt.

• •

DR. MARLIN: When the same thing happened to one of my patients, she called her friends, told them how angry she was that they didn't include her, demanded an invitation to the party they were planning that night, and then went happily.

She basically bullied her way back into the group and was pleased with the results. Another patient thought this was the worst idea she'd ever heard when I suggested it as a possibility to her. Her solution: She cried, got over it, called some other friends, planned a fun event, and decided not to be so attached to the people who neglected her.

Which approach is right? Whichever one—or other solution—works for you. Only you can decide.

LAURA: This has happened to me and it *still* makes me mad. What makes it worse is that it usually ends up being for some stupid reason that you weren't invited. Once I wasn't invited to a party because the whole school seemed to think that I was away.

It's probably the same deal with your friends. If not, then they don't sound like such fabulous friends to me. But the only way to know for sure is to ask them what's going on.

I called up the person I am closest to in my group. I didn't ask outright. I just said, "Hey, did you go to that party?" If she'd acted all flustered and embarrassed, I would have known that my non-invite was a diss and realized that my friends weren't the friends I thought they were.

But she said, "Yeah, too bad you were away and had to miss it." So I knew it was just an honest mistake.

··

I just found out one of my so-called close friends has been dissing me behind my back, saying I have herpes and tried to kill myself. What's the best way to deal?

··

DR. MARLIN: First, be absolutely sure of your sources. If you decide they're solid, then confront her. Say something like, "I've been hearing stuff about me and I know it's coming from you. If you've got something to say, at least have the courage to say it to my face."

The direct approach probably won't change what she is doing. You can only control what you say and do.

But I can promise you two things:

1. If you don't say anything, you are less likely to stop the rumors.
2. Taking action gives you incredible power. You are telling yourself that a few dumb rumors can't reduce you to tears because you know you're better than that and will speak up on your own behalf.

As for damage control, all you can do is go about your life and trust that the people who matter most to you won't judge you by what others say. Good friends will usually give you the chance to explain and they'll trust that you're telling them the truth.

If you persist in trying to speak to them and they still won't hear you out, entertain the possibility that they aren't as good friends as you had imagined. Painful, but it's important to learn who you can trust and who you can't, who is there for you and who isn't.

LAURA: Teenagers, especially in groups, can be outrageously cruel. I think we're all scared that if we don't target someone else, we may be the target.

But the best thing to do is ignore these people. I'm not going to say the rumors will eventually die and no one will ever remember them. I wish that were true, but it isn't. But after a while, if you act cool with it, no one else will care, either. A bad-mouther gets old quickly; no one wants to hear negative stuff all the time. Other people will get scared that the same thing will happen to them. Your close friends will know the truth, and that's what matters. Don't spread rumors to get revenge. It's bound to backfire on you and then you'll look as low as those who talked about you.

....

My best friend started hanging out with someone new and has completely ditched me. I feel betrayed.

....

DR. MARLIN: Your friend isn't betraying you. She's moving on. Unfortunately, sometimes you just have to let friendship shift.

That said, it is often the case that, when you meet someone new who you get on with really well, it's like meeting some guy  you have a crush on—there's this initial brief honeymoon phase when no one else exists. In a few weeks, both people come crashing back to reality.

You could wait around wallowing, but why not use this time to start figuring out how to make new friends? Because even if your old friend comes back, friends are something you can never have too many of.

LAURA: This happened to me, but the other way around. I met this really cool girl at camp and it was like we'd known each other forever. We had the same taste in music, clothes, books, hobbies—everything. A really close friend, who was also at the camp, got really pissed at me because I wasn't hanging with her all the time.

In retrospect, I probably should've been more sensitive to her feeling left out. But one of the reasons we're not really friends anymore is that I felt she was too needy, that I was her only friend, and I didn't want the responsibility. So try and back off a bit. Remember, if a friend starts hanging with someone else for a while, it's not that she doesn't like you anymore or is betraying you. She's just expanding her world and you should do the same.

....

I used to love hanging with my best friend 24/7 because we had such a good time. Recently, though, we don't seem to connect like we used to. What's gone wrong?

....

DR. MARLIN: Time to let things shift.

It happens. You can outgrow friends the same way you outgrow clothes and haircuts—you get older, you change, and you move on to new experiences. And it's most likely to happen now when you're trying out lots of new things and figuring out what who you want to be and what you want from life.

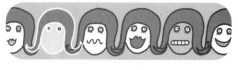

Which may explain why you and your friend no longer click. Yes, it feels like a betrayal—you feel that you're being disloyal by not being all that interested in your friend anymore. What you may not realize is that you may not be the only one who wants out. She may also be bored.

Taking a breather from your friend doesn't mean you have to drop her cold turkey. You can always stay in casual contact with her—calling once in a while or hanging out for a few minutes when you run into each other at school.

But if after some downtime, you still feel distant, be ready to call it quits. And try not to feel guilty. Finding and keeping friends you click with is just another aspect of discovering who you are and what you want in life.

Getting Cool

LAURA: This recently happened to me and a close friend. I don't know if I'm different, or if she is, or both. But all of a sudden, I just felt like I didn't know her anymore. She was joining activities that I had no interest in—like the band and drama club. We had nothing to say to each other. We used to hang after school and then call or e-mail each other every night. Now there were these long uncomfortable pauses.

I decided I had to make a choice: I could keep hanging around her for old times' sake or I could step back from the friendship.

I decided to step back.

That part was easy because we didn't really have that much in common anymore anyway. I think it was probably even a bit of a relief for both of us.

But it still hurts that we're not as close as we used to be. Every day I see reminders of how things used to be . . . there are photo albums filled with pictures of us, I see her at school, the music we used to listen to . . . It makes me sad, but I don't want to pretend that our friendship never existed.

It's hard to accept that we change, even if we don't want to, and that it can destroy parts of our lives that are important to us. But I also know that 10 years from now I am going to have a whole new group of friends and probably a new best friend.

....

My best friend has become such a loser. I'm embarrassed to hang with her. I feel bad ditching her, but I don't want everyone to think I'm a loser too.

....

DR. MARLIN: While true friends can drift apart, the measure of a real friend isn't her popularity rating but how much you care about each other. So ask yourself if you still like her, if you would feel sad if you didn't have her to call anymore, and if you would miss your Friday night movie date together.

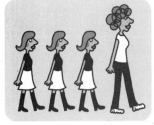

If the answer to these questions is yes, try to stand out and be someone. Be friends with people you like and care about and not people you think are cool. Stop using some stupid artificial rule to decide who you should be friends with. Instead, judge people for who they are.

Of course, for that to work you have to believe it. If you know you're not a loser, you won't act like one and people won't treat you like one.

LAURA: In my experience, a person who is really cool can hang out with anyone and still be considered cool. It's the pathetic losers who ditch friends to maintain some sort of artificial status. So, how cool do you want to be?

10 Things That Really Make You Cool (And They Have Nothing to Do with Who You Hang with or How You Look)

1 Being your own person

2 Being in control of your life

3 Knowing cool isn't how you look, it's how you act

4 Being secure enough to be friends with someone who is an outcast

5 Doing what you believe in, even if others disagree

6 Respecting others when they disagree with you

7 Realizing that everyone is cool in their own way

8 Having the courage to have fun and act purposely weird every once in a while (like talking with a French accent simply because you woke up feeling French that morning)

9 Being able to think, laugh, and have fun without drugs or alcohol

10 Not giving a damn if other people think you're cool or not

Getting Cool

DR. MARLIN'S TIP: Coolness isn't something you're born with. It's a quality you acquire along the way. It comes from how you act toward others. Cool people are aware of other people's needs. They can hear diverse viewpoints without taking them personally or automatically reacting or antagonizing others. They're able to respond in an emotionally charged situation and deal with stress without falling apart.

Friends and Guys

Boys can put friendships to the test. It can upset the balance of a friendship if one of you gets more dates or ends up with a boyfriend. Then there's the question of who your loyalties belong with and where you spend your time. Here's how to juggle all the integral people in your life.

Competition

You can be fairly confident with yourself and still feel envious. Comparison is simply another way to learn about who we are, what we want, and where we stand in the world.

Throughout life, you're going to have friends who succeed when you don't and vice versa. How you cope is a meaningful insight into how you view the world: as a place of opportunity or a place with limited resources where you can't win.

Worry about yourself. It doesn't matter what other people are doing—only what you're doing and what you want. So if you're feeling envious of a friend, think of it as a wake-up call to your deepest dreams and desires, to spur you to try harder and do things better than you have ever done them before.

I made out with a guy I knew a close friend was crushing on and now she's not speaking to me. How can I get her back?

....

DR. MARLIN: Are you sorry? Are you mortified? Was it worth it? Will you ever do it again?

If your answers are yes, yes, no, and no, it sounds like you learned from your mistake. And that's all it was—an error in judgment.

Sometimes, especially when we're feeling down, we pay attention to the *id,* or pleasure impulse, part of our brain (the one that says, "Go for it—it'll make you feel better"), instead of the *ego* (that's the logical part of our brain that looks ahead and sees all the consequences).

That's not to make excuses. As for making it better, gather your courage and tell your friend that the friendship is important, that you know you did a very untrustworthy thing, and ask her what you can do to make it right. She'll be angry for a while, but if you persist in showing that you're sorry without getting frustrated that she isn't okay with it right away, she'll hopefully give you another chance.

LAURA: Okay, it's not like you stole a boyfriend. For all you know, the two of them wouldn't have hit it off anyway. But don't tell her that—I'm just trying to give you some perspective. I know I feel betrayed if a friend buys a shirt she knows I'm saving for. So I can imagine how your friend feels about losing something as close to her heart as a guy, even if he wasn't hers yet.

Getting Cool

The weird thing is that you may not like him at all. It's just that you knew he was desired, so you felt as though you should like him too. And when you got the chance, you went for it.

In that case, you need to keep trying to make it better with her, no matter how much she resists. Be extra nice.

But if you really do dig him, then you have to decide which one is more important to you.

My friend is hitting on my guy. How to deal?

DR. MARLIN: Let her. I know, you thought I was going to say talk to her. But even if you talk to her, you can't watch her 100 percent of the time—and you shouldn't have to. Nor is it likely to change things because she'll think she's having an effect.

And there's no purpose in talking to him. Either you trust him to do the right thing and ignore her or you don't (see Chapter 2).

If she wants to pursue him, what kind of friend is she? And if it turns out he's interested in her, what kind of boyfriend is he?

So start distancing yourself from this so-called friend and then just let it go. Hard as it may be to accept, this one is totally out of your hands.

LAURA: I totally disagree. For one thing, you may be reading the signals wrong. Ask yourself: Is she a super-flirty type anyway?

Also, I think it's hard for any guy—any person—to resist if what you're reading is true and she is coming on strong to him.

So sit her down and shout it out. You don't have to accuse her. She'd probably deny all knowledge anyway. Just probe her on what she thinks of your guy. If she's totally normal ("He's a nice guy and you guys look good together"), then chill. You may be misreading the situation (jealous, much?).

But if she's overly unenthusiastic ("Yeah, I guess he's okay, but I think you could do better") or enthusiastic ("You guys make the best and cutest couple *ever"),* or acts amazed ("Like I could *ever* be interested in him!"), then I'd say she is aware of what she's doing and trying to cover her love tracks. It's not worth confronting her, but I would bump her down to the bottom of my friend list.

And I'd also say something to my boyfriend to make him see her in a new light—something like, "X has no taste in guys. She hits on anything with testosterone. Would you believe she had a thing for [insert name of some really nerdy guy at school]?"

I just dumped my guy. Now I found out my best friend has started dating him. What can I do about this backstabber?

DR. MARLIN: What, do you own him forever? You dumped him.

Okay, maybe he didn't have to date your best friend. But while it feels weird, it's not all that surprising. You and your best friend are probably a lot alike. That's why you're so close. It would have been really nice if she told you she was interested and asked you for the okay (although it sounds like you would've said no). But she didn't. She probably thought (hoped) you wouldn't care because you broke up with him.

Ask yourself why you care so much:

1. Do you want her to hate him because you do? (Not fair—does she expect you to hate all of her exes?)
2. Do you think he's a creep and want to protect her from a lousy relationship? (I doubt it, since you think she's backstabbing you.)
3. Is it that you didn't want him, but you hoped he'd be miserable over losing you for the rest of his life and not immediately dating some other girl, especially your best friend? (See Chapter 2.)
4. Are you worried he'll like her more than he liked you? (He may, but *you* didn't like him, so don't worry about it.)
5. Do you think they're talking about you behind your back? (They probably have better things to do.)
6. Maybe what's really bugging you is that you think she secretly liked him while you were going out with him. (Maybe she did. But remember, she didn't do anything about it until after you broke up with him.)

You can't demand that they break up. But you can still shout it out about how you feel—as long as you do it without attacking her. Remember, she isn't exactly backstabbing you—she just has bad timing. And she may not even realize how upset you are. Try something like, "Even if you couldn't resist him, I wish you felt comfortable enough to talk to me about it first." She'll probably apologize and promise that it'll never happen again.

LAURA: Why is it that girls are more likely to be mad at the other girl? Why not be mad at him? He knew she was your friend when they started going out.

So stop being pissed at your girlfriend just because she was agreeing to date him. Didn't you once like him?

And if she *had* checked with you first, a good best friend would've said, "It's cool," even if it hurt. After all, you broke up with him, you don't want him anymore, and she's your best friend and you want her to be happy.

So let it go and accept them as a couple. When a relationship is over, you can't control who your ex dates next, and he's certainly not off-limits to every girl you know.

LAURA'S TIP: If you do talk to her about it, your friend may offer to break up with him. Don't let her. She'll end up resenting you, especially if you start going out with someone before she does, and you'll end up regretting it once you realize how you are so over your ex you could care less about who he dates (depending on how long you were going out, it takes anywhere from 1 month to 3 months in my experience).

If you're still bummed, look at it this way: She's dating your leftovers.

> My friend's personality has completely changed since she started going out with her boyfriend. It's like no one else exists. What can I say without sounding jealous?

DR. MARLIN: Let it go. Your friend is so happy right now, she has forgotten you exist. But in a few weeks, she is going to come crashing back to earth and the first person she is going to want to call is you because she will need to complain about annoying things her boyfriend does when they're together. Get it? (See Chapter 1.)

If, however, it's been over a month since your friend began revolving her life around her boyfriend, then she may be one of those people who doesn't know how to balance a boyfriend and friends. You can try speaking to her about it—for her sake, if nothing else. Tell her that her boyfriend is really great and you can see why she wants to spend all of her time with him, but her friends are feeling abandoned and they're not going to put their lives on hold for her. It's unlikely you'll get through to her, though.

When girls act like this, it's often because they think that the only way to hold on to their boyfriend is to be with him as much as possible. They're wrong, of course. While togetherness to a point is fine, taken too far (as in not seeing your friends anymore) can suffocate the relationship. The best relationships are those where you make time for each other and make time for yourself.

LAURA: It really pisses me off when my friends do this and it's usually the girls more than the boys. Girls think that they should totally make their lives over for their boyfriends so that they will become the boyfriend's new best friend and he will not need anyone else. Maybe guys don't succumb to ditching their friends as much because they're not as emotionally into their friendships as girls in the first place, so they don't see her having friends as a threat to the relationship.

Getting Cool

I know when one of my best friends started dating this guy that I'm not so fond of, it was like she needed to spend all of her time with him to prove his worth to her life. We'd invite her to things and she wouldn't come if he couldn't make it. So we ganged up and got our guy friends to take out her boyfriend once a week while we hung out with her. She soon saw that their relationship was still strong even though they weren't spending all their time together.

Friendships to Relationships

Crazy mixed-up love feelings often come with the guy/gal pal territory. Sometimes you decide you want to turn into a couple. And when you do, you lose all the things you liked about each other as friends. You get nervous around each other and start acting weird. Or it can work wonderfully for a while and then crash, which can lead to not just the romance breakup but the friendship breakup as well.

On the other hand, because you are friends first you really know each other. Lust isn't the bedrock (though it can certainly grow!). You are really comfortable together, you have trust, you know how to talk with each other, and you make each other feel good. A great foundation for true love that lasts.

I want to tell my best guy friend that I'm in love with him. But I'm afraid that it'll ruin our relationship.

DR. MARLIN: If you suddenly blurt out, "Guess what? I'm crazy for you," he may be so startled that he'll start pulling away from you and your friendship. But that doesn't mean you should stifle yourself.

For one thing, even though it can be potentially embarrassing, you always feel better in the long run when you shout it out because you've taken action and made yourself heard.

And remember, he's not a mind reader—he's probably noticed that you've suddenly been acting a bit weird around him and wondered what's up.

Start with how much you like him as a friend. Add that none of the guys you meet seem to compare. If he says the same thing about girls, you can say you wonder if he wants to try it as boyfriend and girlfriend for a while to see how it works. By putting it in low-key "experimental" terms, it will seem like there's less pressure and give you more room to take a step back and pretend you were just curious about his thoughts.

LAURA'S TIP: Be subtle. This way you can back up and casually change the subject without having stressed your friendship out.

I had a friend who invited her best guy friend over and rented *When*

Harry Met Sally. Then she asked him casually if he thought those sorts of friendships/relationships worked. They got into a heated discussion and ended up kissing by the end of the movie.

If you do tell him and he's not into it, ease your heartache by keeping things to a group situation until you're cool being with him one-on-one again.

Peer Pressure

It can sometimes be tempting to try to bond with people because of what they represent or what they have because you hope some of it will rub off on you. Because you choose your friends and they choose you, you define each other. That means the qualities you use to determine your friends are really telling you something important about yourself.

> I have this friend who never studies and then always copies my work. I hate it, but I feel bad turning him down.

DR. MARLIN: Get strong. It's never easy turning down a friend.

Part of what's making you feel conflicted isn't so much that you feel bad turning him down (although I'm sure you do), but that you're worrying what he'll think of you if you don't help him cheat. Are you scared he'll be mad or call you a goody-goody?

If you feel yourself wavering, consider this: Every time you give in, you're going to get more and more angry with him for using you, more and more angry with yourself for not sticking to your conviction that he do his own work, until eventually you're so angry you won't have any friendship to worry about.

LAURA: Your friend is exerting peer pressure to make you do something you don't want to do. Sometimes you don't even realize you're giving in to

Getting Cool

peer pressure. I remember there was a girl in school no one liked. They'd do anything to see her cry or go away.

One day we were at lunch and she spilled her drink on her pants. I made a loud comment about how it looked like she had peed her pants. Everyone laughed.

I didn't really think anything about what I'd done until I saw the look of humiliation on her face. I realized I was giving in to peer pressure.

My friend Tim has a similar story: "My friends who did drugs never would have said, 'Come on, everybody else is doing it.' But over time they slowly trickled away, and I knew they were leaving because I wasn't joining in." If you don't follow, sometimes people turn away from you.

But is that so bad? Tim didn't think so, and neither do I. Peer pressure is all about manipulation, not friendship. People who pressure you into doing stuff don't care about you; they care about their own power trip. If you follow, that makes them the leader, which gives them all sorts of feelings that they probably crave: power, confidence, security, reassurance that they're okay.

Here's my three-point plan for dealing with the pressure:

1. When peer pressure is obvious, I handle it head-on. I laugh at it, roll my eyes, and walk away. Or, if it's close friends, I say clearly that I'm not interested.
2. When the pressure is subtle, when everybody's doing it, I ask myself, "Do I want to be everybody, or do I want be somebody?" I wish I'd asked myself this question the time with the girl in the cafeteria.
3. When I don't know what to do, I think this: "If I have to be convinced to do something, maybe I don't really want to do it."

Still, you don't have to cut your friend off completely. Instead, offer a compromise by suggesting you two get together to do the homework. This way, you don't come off as a goody-goody or a tattletale.

DR. MARLIN'S TIP: When we think of peer pressure, we always think of it in terms of something bad: smoking, doing drugs, having sex, doing something criminal, getting violent, joining gangs, and so on. We rarely think of the many good ways that peer pressure can influence us.

When it is good, you are a member of the crowd; when it is bad, you are part of a mob. If peer pressure is telling you to do something without questioning why, to do something you know is wrong, or to do something you feel uncomfortable doing, this is bad.

But if peer pressure is telling you to act in a generally appropriate way, to do the right thing when you may not otherwise, or to do more good than harm, this is good. As long as following the crowd doesn't cause you to act without consideration, following is not always a bad thing to do. In a situation where peer pressure is good, individuals in the groups will be acting as individual parts of a whole, each working with the other. A good rule is that if it makes you feel bad, it's bad for you.

> I'm second-generation Chinese and I hate it. There aren't many of us in my school and the other kids act like we are aliens. Some call me Confucius and Chink. I just want to be normal and fit in.

DR. MARLIN: That's racism and it's intolerable.

Unfortunately, we live in a racist society. Which means that there are probably always going to be some ignorant people who seem to need to taunt, tease, call names, or act more violently when confronted with someone who they perceive as noticeably different from them, whether the difference is racial, ethnic, religious, sexual, physical, or simply not mainstream. Think about this: They are often acting out their own feelings of inferiority. They're scared of their place in the world and it's easier to give you a hard time than face their doubts about their own ability to fit in. One sad offshoot of racism is self-hatred.

Unfortunately, answering back won't automatically change the way the kids in your school act. It's incredibly hard to change someone else's attitude, no matter how obviously wrong their POV is.

Lots of minority kids say the key to being accepted is to make your anger work for you by claiming your own identity and feeling comfortable within your own race, no matter what other kids call you.

Getting Cool

Your culture is a part of what makes you who you are; it's something to be proud of.

It'll also help if you talk to someone else about this. Even if you're the only Asian in your school, you're not alone. Try your parents or an older sibling who may have had similar experiences, or other nonwhite students who can relate.

LAURA: Yes, some people are prejudiced, but it's up to you whether you're gonna let it bother you. So forget the "not normal" crap.

If you really want to fit in, then make the other kids fit in to what should be "normal" behavior: treating each other with respect, no matter what your racial background is. Some schools have groups that bring students of all races together to explore their different backgrounds. If yours doesn't, you can start one yourself. Contact the Anti-Defamation League (see "Address Book" on page 257), which sponsors interracial peer workshops. A few of my friends who are minorities got sick of standing out because of what they looked like and decided to make a point by starting a group at school called the Diversity Committee. Anyone black, white, Asian, etc., can come, and they talk about racial issues. It's a really good way for people to learn about others and stop racism.

One Last Friendship Tip from Dr. Marlin

A friend will mean different things at different times in your life. But one thing is certain: The people you choose to spend your time with can have a huge impact on how good or bad you feel about yourself. Who else can you shout it all out to without worrying that you'll be discouraged, dissed, or dismissed?

It's especially liberating when you feel confident enough to move outside your clique, outside your school, outside your age group. We all gravitate toward friends whose lives fall effortlessly in sync with our own. But the best part of reaching out and making friends comes from the chance to gain access to experiences and perspectives you wouldn't have on your own.

Getting
Cool

7
Getting Familial

Your family doesn't understand you. They nag, make you look stupid in front of friends, abuse your privacy, trivialize your feelings. You're right. They don't have a clue.

But they're feeling just as misunderstood, nagged, and unloved as you are. So what's going on?

For the first time, you may see your parents as people who can be wrong. Meanwhile, they're getting used to having a grown-up daughter who doesn't need them as much as she once did.

Many parents find it difficult to work out the balance of power. On one hand, they want to be your friends and not be seen as enforcers. On the other, they want you to have structure.

Brothers and sisters can cause tension as you work out how to relate to each other as adults. You may argue over who is getting more of your parents' love and attention (especially if one of you is going

Eight Things You Wish Your Parents Knew

1 You are thinking things through.

2 You don't want to hurt or worry them.

3 You love them.

4 Sometimes you feel they don't like you.

5 You wish they would assume less and listen more.

6 You want them to know you and be proud of you.

7 You'd like to be sure they mean no when they say it.

8 You wish you could talk with them about sex.

through a tough time and using up their energies). Siblings compete over friends and boyfriends, and often fight about anything and everything.

The truth is it's hard for people, even those who care deeply for one another, to live closely together. With all the ups and downs you're going through right now, the easiest place to dump frustration is on those who, unlike friends, won't reject you: your family. And you see them more than anyone else.

Ultimately, though, if you figure out how to get along with them, you can rest in the knowledge that there is always someone who loves you and who has your very best interests as their priority. Even if it doesn't always feel like it.

Power Struggles

You think they are trying to control your life, but they are probably in a panic. For the first time since you were born, they aren't sure of what you're doing, who you're with, or what you are thinking.

But all they want is for you be a happy, healthy adult who won't spend the next 20 years in therapy blaming them for what's wrong with your life.

> My mother dresses way too young and even flirts with my guy friends, which is humiliating. How can I get her to grow up?

DR. MARLIN: Is this your mother's problem or yours? You're becoming a sexual person, which means she is forced to confront her own aging. She looks like a mom to you, but inside she may feel like she did when she was 20 (I know my mental age is sometimes around 30).

Both you and your mom are now women as opposed to woman and girl. Your mother sees herself as still desirable and wants to be attractive. You see her as a mother and not a woman. If she acts sexual, you feel she is invading your territory.

Don't attack or criticize her. It will only put her on the defensive. Instead, use reverse psychology. Show her how she can look stylish, attractive, and still mature, without trying to look silly and too young. Compliment her on the way she looks when she's dressed in more adult clothes that actually flatter her. As for the flirting, get over it. No one is getting hurt and chances are you're the only one tuning in to her signals.

LAURA: I hate when my mother acts too close to my friends or wears something I would wear. When we went shopping in Express for me, she

How to Fight with Your Parents

There comes a time when you are too old to be sent to your room.

All that most parents want is assurance that you are aware of the dangers out there. That's not being too protective. So give them the five W's: who you are going to be with, what you will be doing, when they can expect you home, where you will be, and why you think this experience is necessary to your life. And call them if you know you'll be late.

found a shirt she liked and I was appalled. This was *my* store. I didn't want her buying clothes there.

Sometimes I think this is her way of trying to stay included in my life. So I just let her do her thing and wear it in a way that I never would.

> My mom is always trying to get me to wear makeup and dress up to "improve" myself. Why can't she just accept me as me?

DR. MARLIN: As a parent who's been known to try to "improve" my daughters and even more as a daughter whose mother tried to "improve" my look (she used to get on my case when my shoes and pocketbook didn't match or when I left the house without lipstick on), I can see this from both sides.

When my mother tried to make me over, I used to think she didn't accept me as I was or wanted to make me into a mini-version of her. Now I realize that she saw something in me—call it inner beauty—and she had her own ideas about how I should maximize it. So try to see your mom's suggestions for what they are—part of her love for you and pride in you.

Getting Familial

Six Ways to Get Your Parents to Let You Do What You Want

1. Build a "trust fund." To make deposits, keep promises, honor commitments, be careful and responsible, and be honest. The payoff is more freedom from your parents.

2. Really listen to what they are complaining about and try to address their concerns with the consideration you'd give a friend who was upset about something you did.

3. Negotiate a trial period. If they aren't keen on your request, suggest you do it on a limited-time basis. Whether or not it works out, when you talk again you'll be prepared to compromise.

4. If you feel hurt, say so; for example, "I am angry and hurt that you don't realize how stressed I am at school." Don't pout.

5. Avoid dead-end lines like "You don't trust me" or "You don't understand me," which only put your parents on the attack. Instead, be specific about why you feel unhappy: "When I'm not allowed to wear makeup to school I feel hurt because I believe I should decide how I look." Offer suggestions or solutions instead of accusations. For example, offer to take off the makeup before you get home.

6. Know when to give up on a lost cause and avoid drawn-out arguments.

LAURA: One of my mother's favorites is suggesting I pull my hair back to "show my beautiful face." She tells me she thinks I'm beautiful, but all I hear is, "You're not like me." It makes me feel that my mother thinks she knows better. When she does that, I just ignore her.

Sometimes she's right, although I hate to admit it. I mean, who wants to admit her mother might actually have a good idea? When she talks to me without giving advice, shows me a picture from a magazine I wouldn't read, or lets me borrow something of hers I like, then I'm more open to her ideas. Especially when she doesn't act hurt if I don't do it her way.

You could ask your mom to send her suggestions this way, too.

My mom and I were having a huge fight and she screamed that she wished I'd never been born. How could she be so cruel?

DR. MARLIN: Parents can say things in the heat of anger that they don't mean. You should try to forgive and forget.

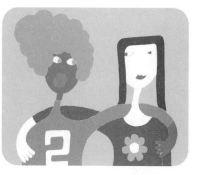

LAURA: My mother yelled once in the heat of a fight that she wished my best friend was her daughter instead of me. She thinks it was no big deal, but it stuck with me.

DR. MARLIN: Actually Laura set me up for that remark. She said, "You wish Robin were your daughter instead of me," and I agreed. At the time I was frustrated and never for an instant thought she'd believe I meant it. Laura's friend, Robin, never has to be pushed to study, and at the time of that argument, Laura's not studying was driving me crazy.

Getting Familial

LAURA: What are you talking about? I *was* studying. And I don't appreciate your no-big-deal attitude. To me, this was a big deal.

DR. MARLIN: So, Laura, if I was wrong (I admit it), what should I do now? What should I have done or not done then?

LAURA: You're the mother, and you should have been able to control what you said (sound familiar?). Second, you should make it clear you don't want Robin as a daughter instead of me.

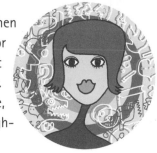

DR. MARLIN: Okay, I'll work on ruling it when it comes to control. There was no excuse for saying what I did. I'm sorry my remark meant years of your thinking I meant what I did not. To clear it up forever: I do not now, never have, never will prefer Robin or anyone else as a daughter to you.

....

My friend and I got caught sneaking out at night and now our parents won't let us hang together anymore. How can we get them to change their minds?

....

DR. MARLIN: You can't get them to change their minds. They are making your friend off-limits because they feel they have lost control. This scares them and they are using whatever power they feel they do have over you. Don't expect instant results. Rebuilding trust takes longer than breaking it. Here's how to do it:

1. Take your punishment and don't complain.
2. Follow their rules to the letter.
3. Talk to your parents. Say you regret your error, point out that your behavior has been spotless since that night, and ask them to tell you what you can do to get back into their good graces. That'll open the door to honest discussion about what they expect from you as a trustworthy adult and you expect from them regarding discipline.

> My father has become so aloof lately. He isn't that way with my brother.

DR. MARLIN: Picture your dad. Now picture a bubble over his head filled with the following items: tampons, bras, mascara, sex-crazed boys.

For your father, this is girl stuff, and he feels that he has no place in your life right now. He may also be dealing with his own changing feelings for you. He sees you not just as his little girl but also as a sexual being, and he probably just doesn't know how to handle it. So he keeps his distance.

Respect his clumsiness. But keep him in your life by talking to him, whether or not he responds. Think about the things that you've enjoyed doing together in the past. Is there anything you'd like him to teach you—how to shoot skeet, how to cook an omelet? Is there something you know he might find interesting—how to go on-line, how to in-line skate?

The more you keep involving him, the more he will come out of his shell when it comes to your girlness.

LAURA'S TIP: Dads like to give advice and feel important and needed, so ask for advice.

I try to connect with my father on his level (talk to him about news or swimming or work stuff), and sure enough, he opens up. It is awkward to talk to him about boyfriends and periods, but the more I do, the easier it is to get into these topics.

> My mother snoops in my things. How can I get her to stop?

DR. MARLIN: Your mother is overstepping her boundaries. But wear the other shoes and consider why she may be intruding. Parents may take it personally that you now want to be left alone. Just a few short years ago, you wanted (and begged) them

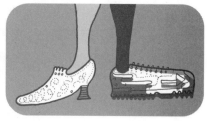

to cuddle you and be with you. They may feel left out and wonder, "What is she doing in there?"

When I feel Laura is cutting herself off, I am tempted to invade her privacy and find out what's going on in her life. Keeping your mother informed may get her to stop snooping.

LAURA'S TIP: When they find something that even slightly confirms their fears, parents are like pit bulls and keep on coming back. Don't give your mother any reason to snoop:

- Hide your stuff in a place she definitely won't look (like where she stores her old clothes).
- Don't bring things like condoms into the house at all.
- Tell her about anything she's probably going to eventually find out about anyway (like a really bad test).

My boyfriend and I were fooling around at my house and my dad walked in. Now my parents are acting strange around me.

DR. MARLIN: Your parents are thinking pregnancy, AIDS, rape. As for your boyfriend, they see him as a sex fiend who is going to use and lose you (see Chapter 3). And now your womanhood is in their face. Listen to what they have to say, and then tell them how much you care about this guy and list his good-boy qualities. Leave it at that.

LAURA'S TIP: Next time, pick a private place to get cozy.

I know a girl whose parents open the door the second she's home from a date so that her boyfriend can't kiss her goodnight. She now makes out on the corner for half an hour first.

I wouldn't flaunt it or make a big deal of it. You are going to kiss and fool around, and your parents are just going to have to face it. What do they think you and your boyfriend do when you're together? Talk philosophy?

Sibling Rivalry

> My sister and I fight over everything these days, even what TV show to watch. We used to be so close.

DR. MARLIN: Here's how sibling rivalry works: You compete for attention from your parents. After a while you are just competing with each other about everything.

I have a hard time watching my daughters fight. I want them to be close and love each other. But then I remember that fighting is an indication of being close—close enough to talk about what you care about, close enough to disagree out loud, close enough to be hurt by the other.

LAURA: Try bonding. Sometimes my sister and I bond over being irritated with our parents—that one always works.

> My younger sister already has a boyfriend and I haven't even had a date.

DR. MARLIN: Getting a guy's attention is at least partly a skill. Since your sister is attracting so many, she must be doing something right. See if there is a way she dresses or acts around guys that you would feel comfortable trying out. You don't want to become her clone or someone you aren't, but there may be a flirty, more fun side of you waiting to be discovered.

LAURA: This is the worst. Guys call for my little sister all the time and I hate it. I hate her for finding the dating thing so effortless. I hate me for even caring about this. I know I should let it go, that there are things I am better at than she is, but it's hard. And then, when I almost can't take it anymore, a voice from somewhere helps me to remind myself: Things change. That guy I didn't think noticed me? He just called. My sister's guy friend has a brother. You never know . . .

Divorce

Just because divorce has become so common, that doesn't make it any easier when it happens to *your* family.

....

I feel like such a freak—my parents are divorced and remarried. Why can't I just have a normal family?

....

DR. MARLIN: You *are* normal. Only 26 percent of American households have a husband, wife, and kids. Half of all teens live in a single-parent family before they reach 18. Families come in many different flavors.

LAURA: I have a friend who lives with her gay mom and her mom's girl-friend. Another friend's parents divorced, married other people, then divorced their new partners and remarried each other. A third friend has so many stepparents, siblings, and grandparents that he's decided everyone he meets must be related to him somehow. I live with my mom and sister and have a stepmother and half sib.

So I don't know what a "normal" family is. We feel like one and so do my friends' families.

LAURA'S TIP: Your family is whatever and whoever you want it to be. Blood doesn't always define it. I feel closest a lot of times to people who aren't related to me. So maybe a family really means being part of a relationship where you feel supported and loved unconditionally. In which case, I'd say my friends are also my family.

My parents always complain about each other to me. How can I get them to stop?

DR. MARLIN: No matter how upset your parents are with each other, they have no right to make you their sounding board. But you have some power to change this destructive scene. Tell them separately how miserable it is for you to hear their diatribes. Try shocking them: "You may hate each other, but I love you both and I don't want to hear it."

After you've confronted them, the next time they start on a tirade cut them off *calmly:* "Too much information."

You can't change how they feel about each other, but you can certainly change how much they involve you.

LAURA: It's hard enough to deal with your parents' fighting without being sucked in. They have people to talk to—that's what friends are for. It's unfair to try to mess up your relationship with either of them.

I thought my folks got on okay, but I just found out they're planning a divorce. I cry all the time.

DR. MARLIN: What you need to remember is this: Once upon a time, your mom and dad met, fell in love, married, and had children. They thought it would last forever. They tried to make it work and then decided to end *their* relationship. They did not decide to end their relationship with you. It affects you, *but it's not about you.*

As tough as divorce is, what leads up to it may be even harder. This is when the war really happens. Chances are you've been dealing with more than your fair share of tense, angry blowouts lately. Now it's finally over.

Many of your friends will have gone through what you are going through. Talk to them about how they felt and coped. Your religious or community center may have a support group for children of divorce (see "Address Book" on page 257).

Getting
Familial

LAURA: My first reaction when my parents told me they were divorcing was to storm out of the living room, screaming at my mother that I never wanted to talk to her again and it was all her fault. I wish I had never said that. In fact, my life and my family's life are so much better since the divorce. You get used to it sooner than you think.

My main fear was that we weren't going to be a "family" anymore. But I still have my parents and my sister; we just don't all live together (which was actually a relief after all the fighting we lived through).

DR. MARLIN'S TIP: Dealing with the breakup of your family is a lot like dealing with a death. You will probably need to ride it out through the five stages of grief (see Chapter 5) before you can cope.

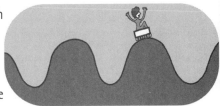

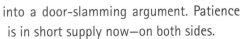

My parents are divorced and I live with my mom. We've been fighting like crazy and I want to live with my dad. He's willing, but my mom says no way. How can I convince her?

DR. MARLIN: The stress of divorce can heighten the normal tensions between you and your mom. A routine "clean your room" can escalate into a door-slamming argument. Patience is in short supply now—on both sides.

As a mom, I wouldn't want my daughter to leave me just because we're fighting. I'd rather have us figure out how to fight. Knowing it's bad enough to make you want to leave may give you both the incentive to figure out how to wear each other's shoes and talk this out.

See if you can stop fighting so much. Create a code word or gesture that signals when things are getting out of control. Cool things down so that you can start tackling what you are fighting about.

LAURA: When my parents first divorced, I would constantly fight with the parent who I was with and say I wanted to live with the other parent. When my parents were together, there was less supervision. So when they were apart, my mom had more time to focus on me and sometimes that would make me feel smothered.

It's easy to think you can go live with the other parent and get away from everything (I still dream about moving in with my dad whenever my mom and I have a blowout even though he's remarried and has a new baby). The fact is that you'd probably fight with your dad too, and he'd also have some stupid rules you didn't like.

···

My parents split up and they're both starting to date. It freaks me out—my dad wears stupid outfits and my mom puts on all this makeup. Why can't they act like parents?

···

DR. MARLIN: Don't dwell on it any more than you want your parents to dwell on your sexual habits. Try thinking how good it is that your parents may find happiness. Which means you won't feel like they're focusing too much on you. The better they feel about their lives, the better it will be for you—now and later.

LAURA: It is kind of weird when my mom goes out on a date, especially when she asks my opinion on what she's wearing. I don't really want to think of her as having the same insecure thoughts I do. I handle it by not getting involved unless she seems to be seeing a lot of someone. Then, just like she'd ask me, I ask to meet him. Not so I can vet him (I wish she'd have the same respect for me), but so I know what to expect.

What I hate more is when my parents lie. My dad used to get dressed up and then pretend he wasn't going out, that this was the way he dressed to stay home and watch TV.

Getting
Familial

> I hate my stepmother! She favors her own kids and treats me like crap. How can I make my dad see how evil she is?

DR. MARLIN: I see three options for you:

1. Keep fighting with your stepmother and remain as unhappy as you are now. You'll grow further apart and end up having nothing to say to each other.

2. You need reassurance that you are still loved. Sit your stepmother and father down and ask for it. Be straight: "Do you care about me? Do you love me? What do you expect from me?" Hopefully, they will answer you as honestly.

   Or you may want to approach your stepmother alone when you are not fighting. As calmly as you can, tell her how you feel about the way she is treating you and how you think you deserve to be treated. She may appreciate that you are talking to her directly instead of going through your father. It could start a dialogue between you.

3. Get some distance. See if you can move in with your mom for a while. I'm not suggesting you run away from the situation, but get some breathing room.

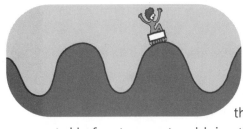

If it turns out you can't ever have a relationship with your stepmother, you may just have to bite the bullet and ride it out until you can get out of the house for good. Some kids think if they are obnoxious, they can get rid of a stepparent and bring their parents back together again. It never happens.

LAURA: My father recently got remarried and he and his wife had a child together. At first, I thought that my stepmother was treating me horribly and treating my new half-brother like the king of the world. But my friends came over and told me how nice my stepmother seemed to be to me. She was trying to be nice to me and make me feel comfortable, but she did have a special connection to her son. That's not to say that this is your situation, maybe your stepmother *is* a witch. But the truth is that your father loves her, and she makes him happy. If you don't like her, you don't have to spend time with her. You can sleep at your friends' houses when it's your father's weekend, or go out instead of spending time with her. When you do have to spend time with her, be on your best behavior; be polite and considerate. That way, if she is horrible to you, your father will see that it was through no fault of yours but simply because she is not nice.

Abuse

My mother hits us hard and often. I'm scared of her.

DR. MARLIN: You have rights even though you're under 18, and every time your mother hits you, she's violating them. I am not talking about the occasional slap or spanking (which I also disapprove of). Physical abuse threatens your development, security, and even survival.

Help isn't far away. Every state has a child protection agency for any child suffering abuse or neglect and you need to report your situation (see "Address Book" on page 255). If you'd rather not call yourself, get someone to call for you. Once you tell someone, he or she is legally obligated to inform the authorities, who will not reveal to your mother where the information came from.

Here's what will happen: Someone from your local child protection agency will be assigned to investigate (this happens in any abuse situation). This person will want to get your story and your mom's story separately, and will also want to interview any witnesses—a neighbor who might have overheard yelling, a friend who saw your bruises. The investigator will put you and your mom in touch with a family services therapist or a court-appointed mediator.

If all other forms of intervention fail, the agency may recommend placing you in foster care, but that happens only in the most serious situations.

When you're summoning the courage to call, keep in mind that your relationship with your mother doesn't have to be this way. Some abused kids get confused because they feel attached to a parent who treats them badly, or they think if they could just be better, the parent wouldn't hit them.

You're not wrong to love your mother, but you are wrong to think you deserve abuse or that it has anything to do with your behavior. It has to do with her own demons.

LAURA: I can act like a bitch and really try my mother's patience. When I'm being that way, I hate myself, but I can't seem to help myself. But it is my mother's responsibility to act like an adult. She can yell or send me to my room, but she has no right to lash out because she can't handle the way I am acting.

DR. MARLIN'S TIP: The danger from this behavior is that upon reaching adulthood you may still assume a victim role in relationships; thus, the cycle continues. Not taking action can also affect your confidence. Studies show children who are regularly subjected to violence by an adult begin to feel a hopelessness that may ultimately translate into suicidal tendencies and misuse of alcohol and/or drugs.

. . . .

My father touches me and rubs against me. When I told my mom, she said I was lying. How can I get her to believe me?

. . . .

DR. MARLIN: *Shout it out, shout it out, shout it out.* What your father is doing is sexual abuse. It often begins gradually and increases over time. Silence allows it to continue, protects your father, and hurts you.

You took the right first step by telling your mother. Though it seems like she doesn't care, deep down she may know what you are telling her is true. But she's just as frightened about it as you are. The truth is too painful for her. And if she really had no idea, well, at least now you planted one.

You must tell an adult you trust as soon as possible—a guidance counselor or clergy member. If it's difficult for you to tell your story, try writing a note or calling an abuse hot line. Your call will be treated confidentially (see "Address Book" on page 255). Counselors will offer advice and support.

Not all abuse is physical. Emotional abuse is extremely harmful. It may take the form of belittling personal attacks: "You're fat, you're stupid, you're ugly"; "You'll never be the success your brother is"; "You're so stupid, I'm ashamed you're my daughter." It may be passive, in that your parents never praise you or make you feel good about yourself.

It may be making jokes at your expense or destroying things that are important to you. It may be constant yelling at you. All these actions can damage your self-esteem.

As a result, you may:

- ۞ Find it hard to make friends
- ۞ Avoid doing things with other people and being places where you're expected to be loving
- ۞ Tend to be pushy and hostile
- ۞ Have a hard time learning or have problems such as bed-wetting or soiling
- ۞ Feel gloomy and depressed, unable to enjoy yourself
- ۞ Become self-destructive, injuring yourself or even attempting suicide

Getting
Familial

One Last Family Tip from Dr. Marlin

If they could, parents would wear a sign that says, "Need us, please, because we need your love." In fact, many parents say their biggest frustration is that they don't seem able to communicate all the love, trust, and appreciation they have for their kids. They want to be involved, so they end up invading their privacy, grilling them about their lives, and attempting to be a part of their lives in any way.

Your parents are confused. They may send you contradictory messages. They may tell you to act like an adult, but they treat you like a child. Before you go out, they may tell you to be good. But then they act as if they don't trust you by making certain people or places off-limits.

The secret to good parent relations is to keep them involved in your life—let them know who your friends are, what your interests are, what you hope for yourself. This way, you stay in control of how much they know and stifle their urge to butt in.

They need to feel needed, too.

8
Getting Ahead

High school can seem to last an eternity. You can't wait to graduate and for your bright new life to begin—the one where you'll finally be free of parents, curfews, your hated English teacher, all those stupid cliques, and the nickname that's dogged you since fifth grade.

Meanwhile, your days seem consumed with tests. Boyfriends. Parents. Parties. More tests. Work. Money. Friends. More Tests. Doing homework gets boring. School activities seem to get repetitive. How can you get excited about homecoming when you've been to a million of them?

One thing is sure—whether you like it or not, you have to spend a lot of time at school. So you might as well figure out how to make it work for you. Think of this chapter as your Cliffs Notes to not just surviving but enjoying high school and getting on with your future.

School Tools

> I hate taking tests. No matter how much I study, I always freeze up and screw up.

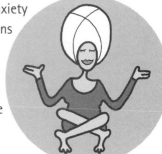

DR. MARLIN: First of all, mellow out. Test anxiety is something everyone has. There are a few reasons people experience test freeze.

If the problem is that you're not prepared and cramming an entire term of work the night before until 3 A.M., it follows that you're going to be too tired to do your best. Here's how to deal:

- ☀ Give yourself a schedule so that you study throughout the semester and keep up with the course work.
- ☀ Ask your parents to keep your favorite fruits, crackers, and cheese around the house for high-energy snack breaks.
- ☀ Get some sleep. Studies show you function at your best with 8 to 10 hours of snooze time a night.

If you're prepared but freak when it's time to sit down and show your stuff, then it's the idea of taking a test that's making you crumble. Here's what to do:

- ☀ Think about all the things you *do* know instead of obsessing about the test. In other words, don't sit there thinking, "I am going to fail." Study.
- ☀ Think of your freak-outs as stage fright: They indicate your work is important to you, which is a pretty neat thing to know about yourself.
- ☀ You might think you need to be a nervous wreck in order to care and do well. But the amount of anxiety you have isn't related to how well you'll do, as you know from the times you've been sure you blew it only to get a 93 (and the times you thought the test was a breeze only to realize later you'd left out a step or two, or forgotten to check misspelling, or added wrong).

- Comparing yourself to your classmates can also kill your grades and sap your energy. Try competing with yourself instead. If you got a B last time, go for a B+ this time. And by pushing yourself to do better, you'll make yourself feel good about your accomplishments. Also, you'll be helping yourself in the long run because colleges like to see improvements in grades as much as they like high GPAs.

LAURA: My friends and I all say we're going to fail before a test, even if we don't believe it. It's sort of an unacknowledged evil-eye thing—if you say it, maybe it won't happen.

I find it really helps if I convince myself that this test is not going to change my life. Also, while taking the test, it's crucial that you take your time. I found that being nerved out makes me rush through to get it over as fast as possible and then I blow answers that I know! Now I take the time to really check my work. (It helps if you read it over like you're reading it to someone really old—that is, *really slowly.* You're more likely to catch mistakes that way.)

If you feel prepared, the test won't seem as threatening. I love to use flash cards. I also find it helpful to talk about the material with friends who are taking the same class.

....
I'm flunking and I don't know what to do!
....

DR. MARLIN: It may seem too late to do anything, but it never is. So have a plan.

First, figure out why you're flunking:

- Do you not get the information needed?
- Have you stopped working in that subject?
- Did you just blank out during the last test?

Getting Ahead

If it's a problem of one score, like on one test or quiz or homework assignment, chances are it's not as bad as you thought. But even if you have lost the whole term, all is not lost. Go to your teacher and tell him or her

12 No-Sweat Ways to Give Yourself a Mental Edge

1 Time of day to take your hardest class: 11 A.M. (when your brain works best).

2 Time of day you should do your math homework: 6:30 P.M. (when you cope best with calculating).

3 Skip the booze. Social drinkers who drink three or more times a week suffer decreased cognitive skills, even when they're sober.

4 Same goes for weed. Smoking pot daily kills your ability to pay attention.

5 Eat well. An extreme low-cal and/or low-carb diet reduces mental flexibility.

6 Studies have determined that students who sit in the T-zone of the classroom (the middle or front of the classroom) tend to do better.

7 The brain takes in information in stages. Taking a 5-minute break from studying every 30 minutes and reviewing every 10 minutes, in addition to a weekly review, increases recall.

that you know you are doing badly and you want to do better. Ask what they recommend. Maybe you can find a tutor or the teacher can give you extra assignments for credit to bring up your grade.

It also helps to outline the steps you need to take to feel like you have a grip. Maybe you need to read more or memorize something or ask more questions. Putting it in writing will give you focus and help you get ahead.

Next, switch your attitude. There is truth in the power of positive thinking. For instance, there was never really a 4-minute-mile barrier.

8 Research shows that people who talk themselves through problems (telling themselves to go slower, be more careful, they can do it) find solutions more easily than those who don't.

9 Exercise. Working out boosts the growth of new nerve cells in the hippocampus, the brain region thought to be responsible for memory and learning.

10 Do a jigsaw puzzle. Puzzles are great brain-stretchers, boosting your analytical skills, memory, and decision-making processes.

11 Read a book in the mirror or wear your watch upside down—this helps stimulate your brain by making you see things in a different way.

12 Take a new route to school—when you follow your usual route, your mind switches to autopilot. But veer off the beaten path and your brain is forced to use its ability to map and make sense of space and direction.

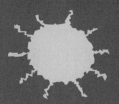

Once Roger Banister beat the clock, many other athletes followed suit because they were no longer convinced that it was impossible.

LAURA: School can be really boring. Half the teachers are bored themselves. The other half have favorites, which is great if you're in their inner circle and horrible if you're not.

The best way to get ahead academically—and also to get a teacher behind you—is to get involved in something outside the classroom. If you're into art, you can join the school yearbook committee. If you're more of the organizational type, get on the prom committee. This will help keep you involved in the school itself and make you look forward to going there. Teachers are also supervising these activities, so you'll get a chance to know each other outside the classroom setting—which may help in the impression you have of each other and make you feel more comfortable around them.

Also, see if you can get extra tutoring in the classes you're bombing in. Sometimes it helps just to get some one-on-one teaching. This really helped me when I could not work out geometry. I didn't become an A student, but I did stop failing tests.

LAURA'S TIP: Borrow the notes of people who do well in the class and see what they think is important enough to write down.

··

I'm not good at anything in school. I want to drop out and start working already.

··

DR. MARLIN: Here's why you should bother with school: An education is the way to get what you really want in life. Think about all the choices offered at school. Besides math, reading, and science, there's art, music, sports, and clubs.

And where else are you going to find so many kids your own age? There are opportunities for you to make friends, especially if you find someone who's interested in the same things you are.

Still, there are some other choices between staying in school and hating it and dropping out.

Know your strengths. Everyone has their own fabulous talents—you just haven't figured out what yours are yet.

Here's how:

☀ Ask your parents and sibs for a short list of what they think you excel at.

- ☀ Ask your friends what they wish they could do as well as you.
- ☀ Really read those teacher comments about your stellar qualities.
- ☀ Check out what comes easily to you and what you enjoy.

Then try shaking up your life:

- ☀ If you're bored or frustrated, sign up for new extracurriculars (choose things that really interest you instead of what you think will look good on some future college application).
- ☀ See if you can study abroad for a year, or try an internship or a vocational school (see "Address Book" on page 259).
- ☀ Think about switching schools. It could be you'd thrive more in an all-girls environment (or, if that's what you're already in, then a coed one).

But whatever you do, don't sell yourself short. A few years back, neither Laura nor I thought this book would happen and now here you are reading it.

So know that things change. You feel crummy and despairing and ready to give up one day, but if you don't, you surprise even yourself with just how high you can soar the next.

LAURA: Besides knowing that school is where my friends are all day, so I'd be lonely if I ever did decide to drop out, just the thought of what the rest of my life would be like is enough to keep me showing up in homeroom every morning.

DR. MARLIN'S TIP: Your academic record doesn't follow you around forever. So you don't have to make the honor roll to succeed in life.

Getting Ahead

But you do have to find out what motivates you. If you're not book smart, maybe you're art smart or sports smart. There are loads of different kinds of intelligence—figure out what yours is (it's the thing you want to do more than anything else in the world) and then enlist your guidance counselor to figure out how you can pursue these interests at school.

Getting In

....

What's the best way to choose a college?

....

DR. MARLIN: It can seem like a lifetime's work figuring out how to narrow your choices of thousands of colleges. But finding the right school is as much about knowing what you want from a college as it is knowing what a college wants from you.

Start by asking yourself *a lot* of questions:

* Does the school have the courses you're interested in?
* What's your budget? (Bear in mind that the cost of living is going to be higher in Chicago than in Scranton.)
* Different colleges also have different personalities. Do you prefer a state or private school, a coed or single-sex school? Does the religious affiliation of the school make a difference to you?
* Be honest: How hard do you want to work? Can you deal with pressure? Check out the median SAT scores of the school's students, the percentage of students who were in the top 10 percent of their high school class, and the number of graduates who continue in higher education after college. The more selective the institution, the more rigorous and demanding its courses typically are.
* What about geography? While many students automatically say that they want their independence and can't wait to move away

COLLEGE APPLICATION CALENDAR

Eighth Grade

✓ Take algebra I and other classes that will help you prepare for college. Find out what courses you will need to take in high school to be ready for college.

COLLEGE APPLICATION CALENDAR

Freshman Year

✓ September: Think ahead—many colleges require 4 years of college preparatory English and math (including at least algebra I and II and geometry), 3 years of college preparatory social studies and science (with laboratory), such as biology, chemistry, and physics, and at least 2 years of a single foreign language, such as Spanish.

✓ September–June: Start on those extracurriculars now. Become a part of student government, school newspapers, an athletic team, a school club, a community volunteer agency, a band or orchestra, a dance team, a youth group at church, or anything that interests you.

from home, there's independence, and then there's isolation. If you're from California and you decide to go to school on the East Coast, start thinking about transportation expenses and so forth.

☀ Does it make a difference if it's a country/suburban or city location (do you want to get away from it all or be in the midst of it all)? Also, remember that a city location will probably be more expensive than a country one. Do you want to go to a large or small college?

☀ Also, styles and cultural attitudes (think liberal vs. conservative) differ from region to region. Make sure you're comfortable with the region's prevailing attitudes and values.

Getting Ahead

You don't need to know all the answers (college catalogs, the Internet, and students going to the school from your hometown can help you get them). But your choice shouldn't depend on just one of the above.

COLLEGE APPLICATION CALENDAR

Sophomore Year

✓ September–November: If eligible, start taking advanced placement (AP) or honors classes.

✓ December–February: Meet with your counselor to discuss what you should be doing now to prepare for applying to college.

✓ March–May: Take the AP tests.

✓ April: Register for the June SAT II: subject tests.

✓ June: Take SAT II: subject tests and AP tests.

LAURA: My mother seems to have forgotten about the social scene, which is a pretty major part of college life. The best way to find out about that is to plan an overnight trip if possible so that you can get a real feel for the place outside the college's PR machine.

Go between March and May, when there're still students around who you can talk to (if you have to go with your parents, try to break away so that you can get an independent point of view on the stuff that matters to you—late afternoon is the time that students are most likely to be around and have time for you).

Taking the campus tour is also a really good idea. It's often given by a student, so you can ask about real things that will concern your life—like the party atmosphere, how to get around without a car, safety questions, the best places to buy health food, if sororities and fraternities play a large role on campus.

Also check out the flyers posted around campus. They'll tell you what people at the school are into and also give an idea of types of clubs, parties, and most popular sports.

COLLEGE APPLICATION CALENDAR

Junior Year

✓ September: Review senior-year course selection, graduation requirements, and college plans with guidance counselor. Register for the Preliminary Scholastic Assessment Test/National Merit Scholarship Qualifying Test (PSAT/NMSQT). Some scholarships, such as the National Hispanic Scholar Awards Program, also base their awards on PSAT scores.

✓ October: Take PSAT/NMSQT.

✓ November–December: Begin searching for scholarships (see "Address Book" on page 256 for Web site aids).

✓ December: Receive the results of the PSAT/NMSQT. Sign up for the February American College Test (ACT).

✓ January: Apply for a Social Security number—it's required on many college applications.

✓ January–February: Sign up for a Scholastic Assessment Test (SAT) preparation course. And start studying

✓ February: Sign up for the March SAT I. Take ACT.

✓ March: Take SAT I.

✓ March–April: Register for May/June SAT I and II (required by some colleges) or the ACT tests.

✓ April: Take ACT.

✓ April–May: Keep an eye out for college fairs at your school or local community center.

✓ May–June: Take SAT tests and AP exams.

✓ June: Take ACT.

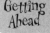
Getting Ahead

LAURA'S TIP: I constantly freak over the college choice and have acquired a secret habit to deal—lots of colleges have WebCam sites. This is a good way to get a handle on a place when you don't have the time or

COLLEGE APPLICATION CALENDAR

Senior Year

✓ July–September: Send away for college applications (call or e-mail the admissions office).

✓ September: Fill in the holes on your resume while you still can. Join clubs, volunteer, and set yourself apart.

- Check with a local high school guidance office, bank, or public library to find a scheduled financial aid night presentation.
- If you need to up your scores, sign up for the October ACT or October/November SAT I.

✓ September–March: If you have not already taken the necessary test, or you need to take it again to improve your score, sign up for, and take or retake ACT or SAT I and SAT II subject tests offered during these months.

✓ October–November: Start working on college applications.

✓ October–April: Start scheduling visits to your top-choice schools.

✓ November: Ask teachers, advisors, and coaches for recommendations.

money to visit. A few independent companies offer virtual and video tours of a large number of colleges.

I also check out school papers, which are often posted on-line and will give you a good idea of what's happening on campus and what the kids are like. The writing in those papers reflects their voice and interests.

- ✓ November–December: Early admission applications due.
- ✓ December: Start writing your college essay (see "Address Book" on page 255 for where to get tips on great essay writing).
- ✓ December 31: Application deadline (the earlier you mail them off, the better).
- ✓ January: Get your parents to compile income tax information and complete taxes early (necessary for financial aid applications).
- ✓ January–February: Get scholarship and financial aid applications.
- ✓ February–March: Deadline for many scholarship and financial aid applications, including FAFSA (Free Application for Federal Student Aid; this deadline is late June).
- ✓ March: Ask counselors to send second report period grades to colleges if this hasn't already been done.
- ✓ April: Acceptances start coming in.
- ✓ May 1: The deadline for most colleges for you to inform them of your choice.
- ✓ August–September: You're off to school. Rent the U-Haul and hit the road!

....

I don't know what I was thinking, but I spent junior year having a good time and getting bad grades. What can I do to get back on track?

....

Getting Ahead

DR. MARLIN: You're still okay. Admissions teams use a mathematical formula to evaluate each applicant's academic record. Your cumulative GPA, SAT score, and class rank are factored together to give you a raw score, which is used to compare you to all the other applicants. They also like to see a trend line of grades and factor in one down year.

In your case, those lousy junior-year grades will drag down your GPA and your class rank. But you can still go for a high SAT score (you have three shots to take it, and the exams are given several times until March of your senior year).

Also, let it shift. Instead of giving up—which is easy to do when you just focus on how you blew it—do what you can to reverse course. Apply to colleges anyway—the worst they can do is turn you down. You may end up on a waiting list or in a less competitive local community or junior college. This way, you can work hard, boost your GPA, and then transfer into the school you really want to go to.

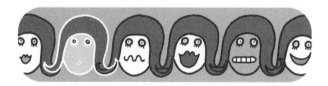

To do this, find out which courses to take in order to make sure the credits will transfer when signing up for courses. You can submit a transfer application in the spring of your freshman year, and, if all goes well, hopefully start your sophomore year at your number one school.

What's the catch? Unfortunately, your high school record will still count. They don't ignore it until you have 2 years of college credit. So you've got to get your grades up right now and keep them up for the rest of the year. Your spring semester grades will figure prominently in your transfer application, so beware of senioritis. Ask your teachers for advice and extra help and/or get a tutor.

LAURA: I feel so much pressure to keep up my grades, do well on the SATs, and just go to school every day and do my homework; it's really easy to let the part of my brain take over that says screw it, I'm doing what I want. To avoid total burnout, my friends and I have devised blow-off days every few weeks. This is when we don't study, do the minimum homework, get out of whatever classes we can, and then hang and do nothing at all. This seems to help us cope until the pressure builds again.

Also, make limits for the lowest grade you'll be okay with. You don't need to always get A's, but that way you won't slack off so much that you stop paying attention.

Show Me the Money

Going to college takes money—anywhere between $10,000 and $32,000 a year. So the more you know about where and how to get funding, the easier it will be for you to attend the school of your choice. Here's your eight-step plan to getting financed, but check out the "Address Book" on page 256 for more details:

1. *Borrow it.* Each year the U.S. government provides over $40 billion in financial aid for students attending college. You'll need to fill out the FAFSA (Free Application for Federal Student Aid) by late June.

   You list the top six schools you're applying to and the schools that accept you send a letter telling how much money you're eligible for from the federal government, state government, and the college based on things like your parents' income and the number of people in your family who are currently in college.

   You're responsible for repaying the loan, not your family. Generally repayments begin monthly within the first year of your graduation. You risk losing your aid if you're making less than "satisfactory progress"—this varies from school to school, but if you're mainly getting D's and F's or going to school less than half-time, you're in trouble.

2. *Go bargain-hunting.* All loans are not created equal. Some have a rock-bottom interest rate (5 percent); others are sky-high (20 percent). Some loans don't accumulate interest until after graduation; others start as soon as you've accepted the money.

   There are also subsidized loans, where the government pays the interest while you're in school (otherwise, you're responsible for repaying the interest that accrues).

   It's important to read the small print and know what kind of loans you have (many of the scholarship Web sites will help). And if you can't make the payments or don't like the rates, you can always try negotiating. Many lending organizations are open to working with you to find a rate and repayment schedule you can live with.

Getting Ahead

3. *Get free money.* Scholarships and grants are awarded to a student to help finance college. In contrast to loans, these don't have to be repaid. Not all are based on grades. Large corporations such as Chevron, Bank of America, and Westinghouse all offer college scholarships, as do many smaller companies. Some universities offer scholarships and loans to students who have done well in a particular field, like math or basketball. Then there's "funny" money—scholarships for bowling, sewing, and duck calling, to name a few. Apply for as many as you can—the amounts vary (some are for $50 and some are for $10,000). A scholarship search Web site will help you find out about these.

4. *Try for the big leagues.* Check out your high school or library's career center for up-to-date information on big awards, like those offered by the National Merit Scholarship Corporation (these scholarships are usually granted to the "upper crust" of entering students, academically speaking), the Educational Communications Scholarship Foundation, the Rotary Foundation, and the Coca-Cola Scholarship Foundation, Inc. Unlike most scholarships, which are school specific, these can transfer schools with you.

5. *Get insider funding.* Your parents' company or labor union, local civic groups and businesses, and your religious institution may also offer scholarships or grants. There are also many organizations offering help to members of a particular ethnic or racial group. You might be eligible for money if one of your parents served in the Vietnam War or Gulf War or emigrated from the former Soviet Union.

6. *Enlist.* The Armed Forces of the United States Reserve Officer Training Corps (ROTC) program fully or partially funds your college education for a commitment to serve in the military for a period after graduation (you have to serve as a reserve officer while in college).

7. *Work for your money.* The Federal Work-Study (FWS) program makes it easier for you to find work on and off campus, since you will be cheap labor (your employer pays only part of your salary, with the government picking up the rest).

8. *Ask the experts.* Once you have been accepted to a college, check in with the financial aid office to see what else is available. Some

may offer awards for students from specific towns or regions. There are also tons of books with information on finding financial aid.

College, College, College

....

It seems like everyone I know is planning to go to college, but I'm sick of the school environment. I want to get on with my life already. Would it be so tragic for me to skip it and try and get a job I love?

....

DR. MARLIN: It's up to you whether you decide to go on to college. But here's a harsh reality: Americans are told they must have a college education if they expect to succeed career-wise in the 21st century. And, on average, people ages 25 to 34 with a bachelor's degree earn $14,000 more per year than high school graduates of the same age.

Still, college isn't for everyone. If you end up working at something that makes you happy, then you probably won't regret your choice. Multimillionaire music and film mogul David Geffen graduated in the bottom 10 percent of his high school, dropped out of two colleges, and went on to work his way up from a talent agency mailroom.

But if you end up shaking the fat off fries at some fast-food joint, you may at some point wish you were still hitting the books. If that's the case, know that it's never too late to return. Colleges often look at you favorably as someone who has gained in life experience.

Christy Turlington spent nearly a decade on the runway before she entered college (she recently graduated from New York University). Katie Holmes deferred her acceptance to Columbia University to star in *Dawson's Creek* (she intends to go back soon).

Getting Ahead

I'm a senior and I know that at the end of the school year I'm going to lose touch with a lot of people I've been seeing and talking to every day for most of my life. I'm scared that when I come home, nothing will be the same.

DR. MARLIN: You're right. It won't be. But part of maturity is accepting change. Some friends will remain friends; others will go their own separate ways, even if you promised to be friends forever. If that's the case, remember that you'll always have the memories of the things you did together and these people helped you become the person you are today.

You could appoint yourself group secretary and keep in touch with everyone in your group via e-mail, phone calls, and letters. But remember too that a big part of going to college is making room in your life for new friends and meeting new people. Staying connected with old friends just for old time's sake or because you're scared of change can stop you from trying new ideas or experiences because you don't want to be seen as different.

LAURA: I don't think it's always as easy to meet people as my mom says it is. You have to put yourself out there and take a risk for a lot of rejection.

When I changed schools and came to high school, I knew no one, and I mean not a soul. I would go straight from school to my room and cry the rest of the day, feeling sorry for myself. But one day this girl in my English class—someone I thought had been in the school for years judging by how many people she seemed to know—asked me if I knew when tryouts were for the basketball team. It turned out she was new too, but rather than run home and hide, she was out there getting involved in clubs and meeting people. She became my first friend.

I also know that when my friends who go to college come home for holidays, they are friendly and happy to see the old familiar faces. I think it's like a trip down memory lane for them and they are glad to be back on their old stomping grounds where they know everyone.

....

I'm starting to apply to colleges. I always wanted to go away, but my boyfriend wants to stay at home and go to our community college for 2 years. I don't want to leave him. What should I do?

....

DR. MARLIN: First, look at the bottom line. Right now you don't want to leave your boyfriend, but you've spent the last 15 years going to school and making an investment in yourself. Somewhere along the way, you formulated a dream of continuing to learn in a new environment. Now you are thinking about throwing all of it away because you don't want to leave your boyfriend.

Let's jump ahead and say you decide to stick with him at home. That means nothing changes. That may sound appealing now, in an I-wish-this-moment-could-last-forever kind of way. But if nothing changes, nothing grows. How will you feel in 2 years if you're still hanging out at the same places, seeing the same faces, and living at home? What will your future look like?

Or let's say something does change—for reasons unforeseen, you and your boyfriend break up. Now you are home living the same old life and kicking yourself for not following your dreams.

LAURA: I have one question for you: Is your boyfriend considering changing his decision and going away with you?

If not, why should you be the one to give it all up? Especially since there's no guarantee you'll stay together anyway. One of my friends could have gone to college out of state but decided to go to college at home to be near her boyfriend. He ended up dumping her, and all she could think about was that she gave up her dream college and messed up her future for someone who ended up not wanting to be with her.

I say go for the long-distance relationship—there's e-mail and you can try to visit each other regularly.

DR. MARLIN'S TIP: Maybe your ambivalence goes even deeper. Maybe a part of you is a little scared over the prospect of leaving home

Getting Ahead

and everything you know. So you hide behind your boyfriend's wishes as a way to avoid taking some risks and going for the thing that you want but frightens you.

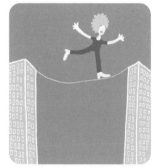

But hiding from your fears doesn't make them go away. Facing them down does. Being afraid of something you also crave indicates how important it is to you: You are facing the fear of failure, loneliness, trying something new, and also the fear that the reality of what you want isn't going to live up to the dream.

··

I'm going away to college and planning to live on campus. But I'm worried about my roommate. What if I don't like her?

··

DR. MARLIN: Remember that there is a difference between "don't like" and "different."

My freshman-year roommate and I slept with the door to our room open and an exit light shining in on us for 2 months until our neighbor asked us which one of us idiots liked it that way. We looked at each other in amazement, each thinking the other did (I figured since her pillow faced the exit door and the light was in her eyes she was probably scared of the dark). We were each too afraid to find out the simplest thing about each other, afraid to offend, to be different, so we ended up being sleep-deprived.

Which is why you should get talking and get a clear understanding of each other's living habits. The most common conflicts between roommates have to do with lifestyle choices—neat freak versus slob, night owl versus early bird. Ask what times she goes to sleep, where she thinks she'll prefer to study, if she's a neat freak. Once you know these things, you can anticipate where trouble might occur and make some ground rules. (Lots of colleges ask for this information on roommate questionnaires, so answer honestly).

Also, give your roommate at least 2 weeks. Everyone is operating under the stress of new things when college starts and it's hard to assess the situation. But if conflict does arise, shout it out ASAP. If you let the situation build up before you confront her, when you do talk, it's likely to end up in a fight and then it'll be harder to reconcile because you don't yet have a shared history that you can fall back on.

The best way to deal is to ask your roommate for a few minutes because there's something you want to talk with her about. The important thing is not to attack. Take uninterrupted turns describing how you all feel about the situation. A statement like "I feel taken for granted when the trash isn't taken out and I end up having to do it each week" is more likely to be listened to than "You're a pig who never picks up after herself!"

Usually a plan of action can be worked out, such as reminders on the fridge as to who's doing what chore that week. Also diplomatically asking if there's anything you do that bothers her can go a long way toward making peace.

You can also ask your resident advisor (RA) for help. These older students are responsible for supervising the peace on their floor and are trained in conflict resolution. If all else fails, your resident advisor can help you find another roommate. If it turns out you can't live with your roommate, don't write her off as a friend. There are friends I could never live with because we're so different in the way we live, but not in the way we think.

LAURA'S TIP: A few of my friends who are in college say it helps if you make contact with your roommate before school begins. Your school will probably supply you with a phone number or e-mail address. So call or drop her a line. Don't try to tell her your whole life story. You've got plenty of time to get to know each other. Just say, "Hello, I'm so-and-so, and I hear we're going to be living together."

You can talk about when you are planning on arriving at school, why you chose the school, what music or movies you like. But don't stretch any truths—remember, your roommate is going to get to know you warts and all soon enough.

Compare shopping lists. Do you really need to buy two ironing boards and two irons? Divvy up the things you'll both use.

This will also help you get friendly, avoid that horrible awkwardness of the first day, and give you a friend from day one.

Getting Ahead

Getting Smart About Earning Money

Part of getting smart is learning how to control your money. It's all part of the same cycle: You need an education to get a good job; you need a good job to earn a good living doing something you like.

Money can represent dependence or independence, personal control, power, security, trust, love, freedom, success, even self-esteem. There is an enormous sense of power that comes from being able to decide how to handle your own hard-earned dollars.

....

I can't spend another summer serving up fries, but I need to earn some money. Are all teen jobs drudge work?

....

DR. MARLIN: Now there are three ways to look at this:

1. Always find work that interests you, so even if the task itself isn't exciting, the surroundings, people, and general purpose of the enterprise will be.
2. Take a job because it's available and the money is good, and then find ways to make the most of it (find the part that *is* interesting, what you *could* learn—for instance, you hate cooking up fries, but like the people who you work with, or the hours suit your schedule).
3. Find a job where the money may not be exciting, but the job is.

The important thing is to get creative. You already know what you don't like. Now figure out what suits you and then build a job from that.

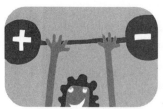

If you love animals, you could walk dogs for a neighbor or start a pet babysitting service. You could also see if any local vets could use an intern. Once you determine what you want to do, use a computer to make yourself business cards with your name, number, e-mail address, and what service you offer. Make mini-flyers and pass them out to your friends, neighbors, and especially teachers and relatives, because most of the time they will be very helpful. You may need to send out flyers repeatedly in order to generate some business.

Also post your services on a bulletin board in a neighborhood community center, school, or supermarket. You might offer free or discount prices to your first 10 customers. The easiest way to get more work is to do a good job and get others to recommend you.

LAURA: Definitely stay away from jobs you hate, no matter how much they pay. It'll just drain you and spill over on how you feel about your life in general.

When I first started working, I got this job cleaning up after piggy adults at parties. It was gross. The clients treated me like scum and I had to pick up half-eaten food that had dropped on the floor and drinks with cigarette stubs floating in them as I listened to bad music all night. I got paid really well and earned great tips, but I hated going to work so much that I never had any energy to do anything.

Now, even though I earn less money doing the office work for a market research firm, I enjoy what I do and look forward to going to my job.

DR. MARLIN'S TIP: Scam alert: The Better Business Bureau (BBB) receives more complaints about work-at-home schemes than any other kind. Beware of any work-at-home offer that requires payments in advance for information, such as assembling inexpensive craft kits or software.

Expensive seminars and training are also suspect, while plans that pay you to recruit others are often illegal.

Get all claims and promises (including details on how you'll be paid) in writing, and if you're suspicious, check with the BBB office in the firm's home city to see if there have been any complaints. Their phone number is in the phone book.

Getting
Ahead

How can I calm my interview nerves? I usually get so freaked going for a job that I can't seem to say what I want to say.

DR. MARLIN: Nervousness usually happens when we feel like we're in a situation over which we have little control. Don't unnecessarily put yourself in an inferior position by feeling like you're at the mercy of the employer to "pick" you. Think of it this way: Even though the employer will take the lead and pose most of the questions, an interview is really just a conversation to determine if there's a match between what you have to offer and what the employer needs.

To mellow out, go to the bathroom before the interview, sit in the stall, close your eyes, and focus on your breath. Force the air out through your nose five times. Then slowly breathe in through your nose, filling your body with cool air. This will relax you mentally and physically.

Taking deep breaths during the interview will also keep you calm. You don't have to be obvious about it. When the interviewer is asking you a question, breathe deeply through your nose. This will also help you to listen carefully to the question and stop you from rushing to answer before you organize your thoughts.

Another way to regain a sense of control is to turn the tables and ask the interviewer some questions. While it's true that you need to impress a potential employer, you also have to decide if you even want the job being offered.

Two good questions to ask the interviewer are to describe what your specific job would be (you may know, for example, that you are interviewing for an assistant position in a lab, but what exactly will you be doing? Cleaning animal cages?) and what a typical workday is like (you'll get a sense of the workload, hours, and how much you'll be working on your own or with other people). Never ask about money until the job has actually been offered.

LAURA: When I interviewed for my internship, I was so scared that I'd say the wrong thing and they wouldn't take me. I tried to prepare what to say before I went in—things that made me right for the job—so that I wouldn't clam up, and that helped. So did keeping my hands on my lap so that no one could see them shaking and also so I wouldn't start absent-mindedly twirling my hair (which I do when I'm nervous).

I didn't get the job, but it was because I didn't have enough experience, not because I was nervous. I think interviewers expect you to be freaked, so they make allowances. All they want is someone who can do the job well, not some cocky kid who struts in and acts like the job should be hers.

LAURA'S TIP: Here, from bitter experience, is what my friends and I found out you should *not* do on an interview:

- ☀ Be late. My work manager says you should actually arrive 10 minutes early to give yourself time to relax.
- ☀ Forget to go the bathroom before you go in.
- ☀ Chew gum.
- ☀ Make mistakes on the application. If you have to fill out an application, photocopy it before you get started.
- ☀ Use a pencil to fill out the application.
- ☀ Answer only "yes" or "no" to questions.
- ☀ Interrupt the interviewer.
- ☀ Avoid looking at the interviewer.
- ☀ Criticize your past employers/boss.
- ☀ Mumble and not speak clearly.
- ☀ Admit that you might not want the job.
- ☀ Use slang or bad words.
- ☀ Call your interviewer by the wrong name.
- ☀ Forget to thank the interviewer for taking the time to meet with you.

Getting
Ahead

What's an internship? Do I really need to do one?

DR. MARLIN: An internship is a great way to test out a job or industry. Although some internships can be quite competitive, generally the amount of experience you need for one is far less than what you would need for a job. The beauty is that you leave with enough experience to land a job. So if your dream is to one day work at a major newspaper, some hot ad agency, or an Internet start-up, internships are a great way to get your foot in the door (see "Address Book" on page 259 for information on how to get one).

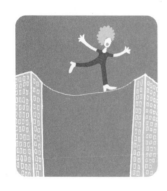

But even more important, an internship, even an unpaid one, can give you all sorts of psychological payoff: confidence in abilities you didn't know you had (you thought everyone could use computers and set up spreadsheets, but your manager can't), a sense of importance ("I've got to get to work or Jennifer won't be able to handle the phones by herself"), a feeling of participation in the real adult world of work ("They pay me to take a lunch break"), and a chance to be taken seriously by adults other than your parents ("My boss used my suggestion and I've only been there 2 months").

LAURA: I'm working as a paid intern at a market research company. It happens that my mother's friend owns the company, so it was fairly easy for me to get the job.

I have never really been in an office environment as one of the workers before, and it's really a good experience to know what office life is like. I see the behind-the-scenes of what makes a company tick.

Although I'm doing the boring stuff (like photocopying and filing), I still feel what I do is important, and that makes me enjoy what I'm doing. Plus I am learning things about the work world that I don't think I would have if I'd stuck with a typical teen job—like how to act professionally, the importance of deadlines, that there are people who really like what they do, and that who you know is as important as what you know, so try not to make enemies.

....

My mother is always going on about how I need to understand money. She divorced my dad and feels she was shortchanged in the settlement because she didn't pay attention to how their money was saved when they were married. But the whole thing bores me.

....

DR. MARLIN: Psychologically speaking, in relationships as in life, money is power. In over 20 years as a therapist, I have learned that, for most people, the only thing as uncomfortable to speak about honestly as sex (and we know how difficult that can be) is money.

Often the person who controls the money also controls the relationship. Historically men controlled more of the money. You do the math . . .

But earning and controlling your own money gives you far more than economic independence and equal say in relationships. Money increases your mobility, your options for saying yes or no, your ability to try new things, your power to make decisions—like are you staying in your relationship because your boyfriend buys you nice things and takes you nice places that you couldn't afford yourself or because you really care for him?

But while money gives you power, it can't buy you happiness or coolness or anything else (although many advertisements would have you believe different). What it can do is give you better control over your life. Here's how: Break down your money into spending, saving, investing, and charity (you decide the percentages).

Spending your own money gives you independence because you don't have to ask your parents for every penny. It helps you to appreciate your purchases more and to learn about the relative value of products (you might think twice about spending $150 on a pair of sneakers when it's coming out of your own pocket).

Saving money is a way of figuring out how to go after your dreams and make them reality in the foreseeable future. Expensive items like a car require budgeting and saving, or you'll never get there without winning the

Getting Ahead

How to Save $1,000 in 1 Year

1 Cut back on small expenses. Rent videos instead of heading to the movies, cut down on your dry-cleaning, and take public transportation instead of driving if you pay high parking fees. Halve your phone bill by calling during off-peak times only. A $3 gourmet coffee every weekday adds up to $780 a year. If you spend $2 a day on junk food in the vending machines, that's $10 a week, $40 a month, and $480 a year.

2 Pay credit cards on time. Credit cards will charge as much as a whopping $35 if you pay just 1 day late.

3 Deduct from your paycheck. The idea behind this one is if you don't see it, you won't spend it. The minute you deposit your paycheck, take 10 percent and put it in an account where you will pay a penalty if you withdraw money (such as a CD), or invest it in your money market account and watch it grow.

4 Keep a piggy bank. It may sound childish, but if you put $3 a day into a large jar, you'll have $1,000 in 11 months. The good thing about it is you can pop extra change in, which helps your savings accumulate quickly. The bad thing is that you might be tempted to pull money out of the jar. And you get no interest. As a result, this method is usually short-term. When you get to $100, make a deposit and get some interest.

5 Pick up extra work. Ask around to see if there's any short-term contract work in your field or take a Saturday job for a few weeks. This is probably the fastest way to raise money; the important thing is to save it.

6 Eat out less, or choose cheaper restaurants.

7 Avoid malls and designer labels. Clothes and shoes are known killers. It's impossible to cut out shopping altogether, but you can reduce the price tags by (a) buying only what you really need and love, (b) shopping around, and (c) keeping away from temptation.

8 Lay off the gift giving. Buy cheaper (but still meaningful) birthday presents. Better still, remember creative gift giving: Make something personal or give your friend that bracelet of yours she's loved forever.

9 Pocket presents. Don't spend the money your grandmother gave you during holidays. Put it out of your reach—a savings account separate from your checking account is a good idea—so that you won't be tempted to spend.

10 Save a fixed percent of every dollar you earn—even if it's 5 percent. Get in the habit now, and just keep at it. It'll pay off.

11 Money tends to burn holes in pockets, so don't carry more than you want to spend.

12 Invest. You can really build your money by investing in the stock market (you'll need your parents' permission if you're under 18). Try investing in things you believe in. For instance, if you love a new computer game, chances are so do your friends and the stock of that company may rise. Think about investing for the long haul—and make sure you get yourself educated. And keep learning. It's your money.

Getting
Ahead

lottery. But say you want to travel for the summer when you graduate—budgeting your money is a realistic way to achieve that goal.

Investing starts you thinking in the long term about the type of future you want to have, including buying a home, starting a business, even retiring one day. The earlier you start investing for your future, the more you'll have, not only because you're putting away a little bit at a time for a long time, but because compounding (the interest you get on your interest) makes your money worth more over the long haul.

Charity is important because part of what money is about is having the means to make the world a better place—and that's everyone's responsibility. Deciding where to donate your money starts you thinking about what you care about in life and helps you realize that what you do really does have an impact.

LAURA: Having control over your own money is more than just earning enough to be able to afford cool outfits. Here's what understanding money does for me:

- ☀ I am able to make more money. I put a part of my salary into a long-term investment account. I've been doing that for 3 years and average over 15 percent! So far, I've made 200 "free" dollars.
- ☀ I can help people. Every year, at holiday time, I decide what charity will receive a portion of my gift money. The charity depends on what I'm interested in. Donating makes me feel a part of something that I believe in.
- ☀ I know how to save for things. Last year, I really wanted these boots my mother said I didn't need. I put money aside and I'm looking at them on my feet right now.

LAURA'S TIP: Figuring out how to manage money doesn't have to be boring. I like logging on and pretending to invest with on-line games like Mainxchange (www.mainexchange.com), which allows you to sink $100,000 of virtual currency ("bux") in real-life stocks like McDonald's or The Gap. If the stock does well, you could win prizes.

There are also magazines geared for teens like *Young Money Magazine*, which make talk about saving money interesting.

Or you could get interested in interest rates (the rate that can determine how much you earn on your savings and also how much interest you pay back on credit-card and college loans) by joining the Fed Challenge, an annual economics competition for high school students sponsored by the Federal Reserve Bank.

Or you could become a Life, Payday, or Monopoly champ.

One Last Getting-Ahead Tip from Dr. Marlin

The thing to remember is that very few people are all-around whizzes. We possess many different types of intelligence in varying degrees. You may be very logical (science smart), be sensitive to others' moods and feelings (people smart), enjoy reading and writing (language smart), enjoy working physically (body smart), have a good ear (musically smart), feel most at ease with pictures and images (visually smart), and so on.

Here is how to figure out what your own particular brand of potential is:

* Chart it. Try tapping into your childhood dreams. These fantasies reveal your passions and talents in their purest form. What did you most love doing, say, 5 years ago? The answer can tell you much about your aspirations and motivations.

   The same goes for thinking about what activities outside school give you satisfaction. Maybe you love caring for animals or organizing parties. These skills can be as important as getting an A in algebra.
* Organize. Plan an ideal day for yourself. How would you spend your time if you had no money worries, no time constraints, no outside responsibilities? All of these are clues to what makes you tick.

Getting Ahead

☀ Find a role model. Find a mentor—essentially a savvy fairy godmother or godfather (or several) who will guide and advise and won't be critical.

Surprisingly, teachers are more likely to fit this bill than parents (especially if your parents aren't behind you 100 percent). If a particular idea gets your pulse racing, let your teacher know. Talk to them after class and ask what books you can read or things you can do to delve further into whatever subject interests you. Take advantage of any adult who can make suggestions about how to pursue your passion and steer you to other supporters and resources. For instance, maybe your second cousin works at a radio station and you're interested in journalism. Pick up the phone! These people can stimulate, challenge, and encourage you.

☀ Reverse your thinking. Stop thinking, "I'm going to fail." Like I said, there are all different kinds of smarts. Yours may not be the academic kind. If you rarely get higher than a D in the three R's but have success or interests in other areas, focus on and excel in these.

A Final Life Tip from Laura

I always thought of myself as a dork. I thought I was the only self-conscious girl in the world, and that I was weird and an outcast. I have made my share of mistakes, and there's so much that I wish I could change. I always thought that everyone else just knew how to handle life better than I did. I was scared of everything from thunderstorms to shots, and had tons of panic attacks. But I came to realize that I'm not weird—I'm normal.

We're all concerned with how others view us. It's the ones who hide it well who are considered to be cool. Looking at my younger sister and her friends now, I can see how even the coolest girls in her class are looking at everyone else to see what they're doing so that they don't look weird. For instance, I noticed something about the girl who is supposed to be the most confident and the most popular in her grade: When this girl is at a party and wants to dance, she looks to see if everyone else is dancing and how they're doing it so that she can dance like them. She's just as afraid of standing out and being thought of as different or weird.

It took me too long to realize that feeling awkward and insecure is normal, and I wasn't weird. There was nothing for me to feel self-conscious about. I finally realized that I should embrace my differences and walk with my head up. Writing this book has given me perspective on life as a teenage girl. I am now more aware of the feelings girls have, and I realize that the girls I was so jealous and afraid of when I was younger are not really all that great. They had confidence on the outside, but our insecurities and concerns were not so different on the inside.

Someone once told me that when guys look in the mirror, they block out what looks bad and concentrate on what looks good. On the other hand, when girls look in the mirror, they concentrate on what's wrong with them. It's no wonder guys are so confident and think that they can have anything they want. They can, because they have the attitude. Take a lesson from the guys. Decide that you like who you are, and if you give off that attitude, others will like you too. Everyone is different, everyone has things that they hate about themselves (even guys); it's completely normal. But the trick is to embrace the differences instead of shying away from them. Not only will people respect and like you more, but you will be proud to be you, which is the most important life lesson of all.

A Final Life Tip from Dr. Marlin

Laura and I wrote this book because we believe girls should feel proud of their unique interests and ideas, of their differences from boys and from each other.

It's tough thinking that you are the only one who thinks or feels or looks a certain way. You might be hard on yourself for not being like everyone else, or you may be getting flak from other (less secure) individuals for not conforming to the status quo (as if this is

Getting Ahead

Laura's Eight Things That "I Wish I Had Known Earlier"

1 Grades only matter for now and getting in to a good college (and scholarships for paying for that college!).

2 Keeping your mouth shut usually hurts you.

3 Do what you really want to do rather than have regrets for the rest of your life.

4 Being shy won't get you anywhere, and being outgoing won't kill you.

5 What you eat actually does matter—a healthy diet gives you the energy to do the things you want in life.

6 Family isn't something to be ashamed of—they're the ones who usually stick with you no matter what.

7 *Everyone* is self-conscious.

8 Things change. So just because life sucks at one moment doesn't mean it always will.

the most important thing). But fast forward to the future: How much of the crowd you are or aren't part of now has nothing to do with your place in the real, adult world.

Remember, normal is a relative term. What your group, culture, and times deem weird, might be normal elsewhere, whether among a different clique or in another land. And you are constantly changing as your options and explorations broaden, so give yourself permission to decide for yourself what is weird and what is normal. After all, normal is just shorthand for trying to fit in. Of course we all want to be a part of our world—and of course we all want to be spe-

Dr. Marlin's Eight Things "I Wish Someone Had Told Me When I Hit Adolescence"

1 Life is not as hard as everyone says it is.

2 It's not as tough to make friends as you might think. A lot of people are actually pretty lonely and are thrilled when you make an effort to get to know them.

3 Sometimes you are not going to have a clue as to what's going on. That's okay. Just don't be afraid to ask questions; usually no one else knows what's going on, either.

4 Being independent is fun—but it's also stressful. You finally are the only one who is responsible for you.

5 To do well, you are going to need to study/work 100 times harder than you did last year.

6 Doing your work, eating decently, and keeping some order in your life may seem too conventional for your lifestyle, but it will help you feel in control.

7 What you've done or who you've been in the past doesn't matter.

8 You can work really hard on an assignment and still do poorly.

Getting Ahead

cial. The trick is to keep working at the balancing act in a way that works for you.

Lastly, getting cool means getting what these years are about: figuring out what excites you and what makes you scared and then using that knowledge to challenge yourself to become a strong, independent person. Part of the process is testing your ideas and opinions to develop your own voice (journaling, starting your own zine or band, fighting for a cause), deciding upon your belief system (religious, political, moral), participating in your community (volunteering, becoming ethnically/racially involved, performing random acts of kindness toward strangers).

Because if you're truly cool, you know that even though you may not feel or think the same way a few years from now—or even tomorrow—how you treat the world and yourself right now is, ultimately, what will help you break out of any stultifying stereotypes and become your own, best person.

Life is the details, the small moments, when you make a decision for yourself and realize you can take care of yourself. It's in that instant you really see the look on someone's face and connect with them. It's in accepting the truth and negotiating life's bumps. It's in learning to handle your emotions—instead of yelling, you try to understand. And it's in seeing your parents, your teachers, and your friends as separate, whole people who have their own lives, their own fears, their own hopes.

Think of this book as a caring guide to help you determine what kind of relationships, education, career, goals, values, beliefs, status—what kind of life you want.

It's up to you to take it from here. We're rooting for you!

Address Book

Abuse (Family)

National Child Abuse Hot Line (800-4-A-CHILD) will help if you've been physically or sexually abused.

Abuse (Relationship)

Safe (800-799-SAFE) is a hot line for dating-violence victims. Counselors will give you advice about safety and refer you for ongoing help in your area

Allies/Counseling

Boys Town National Hot Line at 800-448-3000 (24 hours) works with children and families in crisis.

Youth Crisis Hotline is a 24-hour crisis hot line and information and referral for youth with parent problems (800-HIT-HOME; www.1800hithome.com).

Girls Incorporated (www.girlsinc.org/) is a national youth organization dedicated to helping girls become strong, smart, and bold.

Students Against Destructive Decisions (SADD) is run by teens to help students make the right decisions concerning underage drinking, DWI, drug abuse, and other difficult decisions (SADD National Box 800, Marlboro, MA 01752; 800-787-5777; www.saddonline. com/).

Sisters International, Inc., is a nonprofit organization to help develop women as leaders in the family, workplace, and community (P.O. Box 2188, Portland, OR 97208-2188; 503-645-8326; e-mail: corp@sisters-international.org; www.sisters-international.org).

NineLine at 800-999-9999 (24 hours) is a nationwide crisis hot line for youth needing help dealing with issues like drugs, domestic violence, and sexual abuse.

College/Financial Aid/Scholarships

The Common Application (www.commonapp.org) is a form that is currently accepted by 195 colleges (it also includes tips on applying and picking colleges). Students fill it out once, then mail copies to all the schools to which they are applying. Schools that have two-part applications will mail out a supplemental form after receiving the Common Application.

CollegeGate (www.collegegate.com/) is an essay editing service offering 100 free sample essays, free essay writing tips, and a college search engine.

CollegeNET (www.collegenet.com) lets you enter your specific criteria (school size, tuition, sports programs, etc.) and draws up a list of matching schools. Or you can browse through their database state by state.

CollegeView (www.collegeview.com) gives you a virtual tour of various colleges.

The College Board (www.collegeboard.com) sponsors the SATs and PSATs and offers sample SATs, test-taking tips, and software you can buy to practice with. Plus you can register on-line to take the exams.

The Princeton Review's *The Complete Book of Colleges,* the College Board's *The College Handbook,* and *Cash for College: The Ultimate Guide to College Scholarships* by Cynthia Ruíz McKee and Phillip C. McKee, Jr. (Quill) have solid information on university and college statistics.

The Smart Student Guide to Financial Aid (www.finaid.org) offers information on financial aid and includes a free scholarship search.

Free Application for Student Financial Aid (FAFSA) is your one-stop government financial aid shopping site (800-433-3243; **www.fafsa. ed.gov**).

Depression

National Mental Health Association (**www.nmha.org**) offers on-line depression screening.

National Suicide Hotline: 800-SUICIDE (800-784-2433).

Discrimination

If you think you are a victim of discrimination, contact the Office on Civil Rights (800-368-1019).

Anti-Defamation League sponsors interracial workshops (823 United Nations Plaza, New York, NY 10017; 212-490-2525; **www.adl.org**).

Divorce

Family, Assessment, Counseling and Education Services (FACES Inc.) is a nonprofit organization whose purpose is to provide help for children experiencing the grief of their parents' divorce (1966 E. Chapman Ave., Ste. G, Fullerton, CA 92831; 714-879-9616; www. facescal.org/).

Drugs/Alcohol

Address Book

National Clearinghouse for Alcohol and Drug Information has information on alcohol, tobacco, and drug abuse and prevention. Referrals to treatment centers, research, groups, information on drugs in the workplace, community programs, and AIDS (800-788-2800; e-mail: info@health.org; www.health.org).

www.clubdrugs.org is a source for information on MDMA (Ecstasy), GHB, Rohypnol, ketamine (Special K), methamphetamine, and LSD.

Teens Against Drugs/Community Outreach Program (TAD/COP) combines drug education with drug-free activities like concerts, carnivals, sporting events, and camping trips. The staff will help you set up a program in your community (261 Yvonne Ave., Crossville, TN 38555; 931-456-2859; www.tadcenter.com).

Alateen is a national organization (with meetings in all 50 states) for young people who have a relative or loved one with an alcohol problem (888-4AL-ANON; www.al-anon.org).

Eating Disorders

Eating Disorder Recovery Online provides services and important information to assist people exhibiting characteristics of disordered eating (888-520-1700; e-mail: jrust@edrecovery.com; www.ed recovery.com).

Smash! (www.dandyweb.com/smash/smash.html) is committed to creating positive body images for all races, religions, ages, and sizes of women.

Grief

Grief Net (griefnet.org/) is an Internet community of persons dealing with grief, death, and major loss.

Internships

New InternshipPrograms.com (www.internships.welfleet.com/home. asp) lists hundreds of internship opportunities.

National Internships Online (www.internships.com) regularly updates its extensive list of internships.

Mental Health

Anxiety Disorders Association of America (ADAA) offers information and advice (11900 Parklawn Dr., Ste. 100, Rockville, MD 20852; 301-231-9350; www.adaa.org).

Parents

Youth Crisis Hotline is a 24-hour crisis hot line and information and referral for youth with parent problems (800-HIT-HOME; www.1800hithome.com).

Puberty

Virtual Kid Puberty 101 (www.virtualkid.com) covers all the changes your body is going through.

Rape

The Rape, Abuse & Incest National Network (RAINN) operates a national toll-free hot line 24 hours a day. It will automatically transfer you for free to the rape crisis center nearest you, anywhere in the nation. The organization also offers free confidential counseling (800-656-HOPE; e-mail: RAINNmail@aol.com; www.rainn.org).

Running Away

National Runaway Hotline (800-231-6946) is a 24-hour message relay service to parents as well as a help line for runaways.

Self-Mutilation

SelfHarm.Com (www.selfharm.com/) offers information about self-harming behavior, self-injury, self-mutilation, self-abuse, and cutting, plus coping skills, alternatives to self-injury, support groups, personal cutting stories, and ways to stay safe.

Address
Book

Sexuality

Condomania (www.condomania.com) sells a wide variety of condoms as well as offers general information on latex protection.

Planned Parenthood offers balanced sexual counseling and emergency contraception and abortion information (800-230-PLAN will automatically connect you to the center nearest you; www.planned parenthood.org/).

Planet Out (www.planetout.com) is a good place to connect with other gay youths.

National STD Hotline has information on minor and major STD infections (including yeast, chancroid, herpes, genital warts, syphilis, and gonorrhea), as well as referrals, information on prevention, and free pamphlets (800-227-8922; www.ashastd.org/).

HIV/AIDS Teen Hotline (800-440-8336) and Teens Teaching AIDS Prevention (800-234-TEEN) are staffed with teens who can answer questions, make referrals, or just talk.

Spirituality

Finding God in Cyberspace (www.fontbonne.edu/libserv/fgic/fgic.htm) is an impartial resource for exploring different religions on-line.

Sports/Fitness

For a free fitness profile, log on to www.homearts.com/depts/health/ffindf1.htm.

The Women's Locker Room (www.fitnesslink.com) is a motivational site for working out.

Get a free Morphover (www.efit.com). Just register and send a digital photo. They rejigger it using your body type and size to show you what you'd look like if you exercised and ate right.

Women's Sports Foundation answers questions on sports and physical fitness for women (800-227-3988; e-mail: wosport@aol.com; www.womenssportsfoundation.org).

Stepfamilies

Stepfamily Foundation helps you and your family cope with your new relationship (333 West End Ave., New York, NY 10023; 212-877-3244; www.stepfamily.org/).

Stress

Get time-management tips on-line at www.mtsu.edu/%7Estudskl/tmths.html.

Index

Index

Index

Index

Index